# OPERATION *Daughters* ADDICTED

# OPERATION *Daughters* ADDICTED

## Positive Strategies to Overcome the Dual Addiction of Eating Disorders and Substance Abuse

BY

SANDY MULLEN
AND
CATHY NAPIER

FOREWORD BY NAOMI JUDD

INKWATER PRESS
PORTLAND • OREGON
INKWATERPRESS.COM

Cover and interior design by Masha Shubin

Girl Eating Drugs © Isakovich Alina. BigStockPhoto.com



Publisher: Inkwater Press | www.inkwaterpress.com

Paperback
ISBN-13 978-1-59299-797-8 | ISBN-10 1-59299-797-X

Kindle
ISBN-13 978-1-59299-798-5 | ISBN-10 1-59299-798-8

Printed in the U.S.A.
All paper is acid free and meets all ANSI standards for archival quality paper.

1 3 5 7 9 10 8 6 4 2

# Table of Contents

# Foreword

In recent years, there has been increasing concern among medical professionals about the epidemic problem of eating disorders and chemical dependency, especially as these disorders afflict women. The image of anorexic, stick-thin models and other celebrated figures in the entertainment industries is often blamed for a heightened anxiety and dissatisfaction among young women obsessing daily over their own body image.

The media continues to report on their numerous problems, substance abuse and their trips to rehab and legal problems. The public sees the devastating effects that eating disorders and chemical dependencies may wreak on the very celebrities that have been so idolized. There have been many stories of the terrible toll that these diseases have taken on the careers and, indeed, the lives themselves, of public figures. More and more frequently, people everywhere are realizing that they must seek treatment if they are to become whole and well again.

Unfortunately, with all the best intentions, so many of those who enter into treatment programs, either on their own or with the encouragement of family and friends, are returning to their former lives and resuming the habits that brought them into treatment in the first place. Soon they find themselves back into treatment. The treatment programs them-selves become "a swinging door," when the individuals core issues aren't identified and dealt with.

The fault may lie to some extent with programs which, historically, tend to regard eating disorders and chemical dependencies as separate and distinct problems, to be dealt with individually and with different methods. Cathy Napier and Sandy Mullen, in this book *Operation Daughters Addicted,* have recognized that these two disorders very often are closely related: Eating disorders, drug and alcohol abuse, Cathy and Sandy demonstrate, have become dual dependencies.

Take for example the case of a woman who seeks treatment for an eating disorder, whether it is over-eating, bulimia, or anorexia. She may have discovered along the way that pills, in the form of amphetamines or opiates such as codeine compounds, or even alcohol, can reduce or almost entirely eliminate her appetite. She loses weight but in the process has acquired a chemical dependency—a "hidden addiction."

Or, in another case, a woman with a drug or alcohol dependency may discover that she is losing weight by virtue of her loss of appetite. To maintain what she considers a more attractive figure, she may then begin reducing her intake of food and nutrients to the point that she acquires, in addition to her chemical dependency, a full-blown eating disorder. In both cases, the patient who has been treated for one disorder returns to treatment in the throes of the other disorder.

Cathy and Sandy came upon their unique insight into the little understood phenomenon of dual dependency through years of professional practice and clinical work in their individual specialties: Cathy as a therapist treating chemical dependency and Sandy as an R.N. treating eating disorders. Puzzled by the failures of otherwise excellent programs, the two began comparing notes and observations and discovered that treatment of one addiction, while apparently successful, was in fact feeding the growth of another, hidden addiction.

This collaboration is the result of their discoveries and the joint effort to treat their patients for more than one addiction simultaneously. In these pages, Cathy and Sandy tell the brutally honest personal stories of a number of dually addicted people who they have treated, then take the reader through the processes by which their patients achieved awareness of the presence and dangers of the hidden addiction, and describe paths taken by these people to total recovery.

*Operation Daughters Addicted* is written as if spoken to the individual reader, in a conversational and non-technical style. The reader is drawn into forging a path to her (or his) own recovery through a series of clearly defined steps leading to increased self-awareness and commitment to succeed. Readers are invited and guided to write their own stories by way of simple exercises offered at the end of each chapter. Additional exercises provide a spiritual component, which, at the reader's option, provide guidelines to calming prayer or other beneficial meditations.

This is where I brag that Cathy is one of my oldest and dearest friends. She's been an empathic, smart gal since she was small. Cathy and Sandy describe their own battles with, in one case, alcohol/pills, and in the other, an eating disorder. This book is the result of Cathy's lifetime commitment to helping others.

Cathy and Sandy acknowledge that addiction is a family disease. I personally was grateful that Cathy and Sandy acknowledged that addiction is a family disease. My own two daughters, Wynonna and Ashley, have sought help. Wynonna battles an eating disorder and Ashley has suffered major depression. The family chapter gives family members practical tools for dealing with resentments and regrets that accompany dependencies and make it clear that family genetic make-up as well as family dynamics become a part of the battle. They illustrate how an entire support system contributes to getting the disease into recovery.

Cathy Napier and Sandy Mullen are to be congratulated for their work in bringing this secret of dual addiction to the forefront. They bravely expose the lethal combination of the two killer diseases and are to be commended for encouraging the treatment community to treat patients for both diseases simultaneously. *Operation Daughters Addicted* offers entirely new insight into what has been until now a largely unrecognized phenomenon and gives the reader both renewed hope and tools that enable him or her to find the joys of life free of dependencies.

Naomi Judd

Singer, Author and Motivational Speaker 2012

# Authors' Note

This book began in the disappointing experience of seeing our patients leave treatment on the road to recovery, only to witness them returning to treatment a few months later, worse off than when they left. We had become frustrated as professionals by the prevailing protocol by which it was believed that addictions should be treated one at a time. Happily, when the treatment team decided to prescribe chemical dependency treatment along with the eating disorder treatment for patients, we started to see patients getting into full recovery. After many years of keeping track of those we had treated for their addiction to and abuse of chemicals as well as their addiction to food, we began to see and then document successful long-term recoveries. The results that we witnessed, the testimonies of our patients, and the insights we gained, we now pass along to you in this book. Since have had our own battles with addiction, we felt that teaming together would give us more insight to the protocol for life-long recovery for our patients. We both have a desire to see the eating-disorder patient and the chemical dependency/abuse patient achieve a life of quality without bondage. We believe that anyone who suffers from mental illness, whether it is depression, anxiety, or addiction, can benefit from the tools we have provided the reader.

# Acknowledgments

In the course of this journey, there have been many fine professionals whose work I, Sandy, am proud to acknowledge. Individuals from whom I have a great sense of support, include the R.N.'s Kathy Aferiat, Nancy Park, Jeri Zenwinski, Cindy Short and Susan Mendoza. The therapists include Kim Rockwell-Evans, Cynthia Hutchinson, Gloria Dean, Jim Harris, and Pam Jenkins. Dietitians include Carla Schattle, Carol Park, and Jean Bivona. Art therapists Teresa Jackson, Betty Keller, Susan Merecle, and Abby Kalish were an amazing group of women to work with, as were psychiatrists Dr. Urusla Kelley, Dr. Yaprac Harrison, and Dr. Margaret Miesch. I send a special thanks to Jim, my husband, who has always encouraged my writing efforts and has been my biggest fan, and I send special love to my three wonderful sons.

Throughout the 34 years that I, Cathy, have worked in the mental health field, I have had the privilege of being associated with many intelligent, gifted, and caring professionals. I would like to acknowledge therapists, physicians, and support staff, who have worked alongside me. Tip Mckay, Mike Gaffney, Dr. Stephanie Darsa and the support of psychiatrists Dr. Laurie Klieman, Dr. Chreyé Callagahan, Dr. John Wilson and the late Dr. Mary Conrady. My co-workers, Amy Pool, George Kane, Jim Kennedy, Joyce Zang, Debra Singer-Hanson, Chuck Hanson, Eugenia Vasquez, Barb Shannon, Rose Whitcomb, Dr. Alice Crawford, Cathleen Weidner, Horace Whitfield, Suellen James, Dennis Reinecker, Dr. Jon Crook,

Dr. Sharon Clark, Dr. Michael Jarrard, Bill Holtmeyer, Dr. Quinella Minix. Ron Hesslein and to Susan Winn for their support to the Burlington Northern Santa Fe Railway Employee Assistance Team. Kevin Vaudt, Medical Field Manager with Burlington Northern Santa Fe. Amanda Gambrell and Rick Foley who are dedicated to the cause of helping employees of the Burlington Northern Santa Fe Railroad maintain their physical and behavioral health. I give special thanks to my mentor, Dr. Leslie Secrest the Chair of Psychiatry at Presbyterian Hospital of Dallas. Thank you to my good friend Dina Horneffer who would gently listen to me during the frustrating times. Naomi Judd my loyal friend for 56 years. With thanks too to our editor, Erika Cooper, for her patience with us and her belief in this book. Finally, I reserve my greatest gratitude for my wonderful daughter, Holly, who has always been my motivation in life and to the people of Israel who held me up through the tough times.

# Preface

For more than 15 years, I have had the privilege of working with Sandy Mullen, R.N. in an inpatient psychiatric and addiction unit. We groped our way, learning as we went, developing our program and treating our patients.

As the body of knowledge evolved over the past 20 years, it became increasingly clear that it is critical to treat addictions simultaneously and in an integrated way. To be successful, a balanced treatment approach must be comprehensive, through an evaluation (physical and psychiatric) with appropriate treatment plans that include medications, education, a therapeutic milieu and a strong 12-step orientation. A strong family component must also be implemented. Sandy and Cathy have developed a book that describes how the patient and family can achieve wellness through all the above mentioned treatment protocols. I applaud their good work.

R. Lynn Markle, M.D.

Psychiatry
3609 Cedar Springs
Dallas, Texas 75219

When we first began working with eating disorders, little did we know how widespread our knowledge would have to be in order to address this serious life endangering disorder that sounds so benign. We quickly discovered that we needed knowledgeable internists, cardiologists, gynecologists, and endocrinologists at our sides, as well as people who understood addictions. We discovered the need for family therapy and for the need of authenticity. Our patients were coming from families that kept secrets and we recognized the importance of establishing a staff that focused on honesty and openness. These two strong capable women, Sandy and Cathy, with their many years of clinical experience, have been willing to take the time out and put on paper their discoveries about what works and what doesn't work in the treatment of eating disorders. I am thankful for their generosity in sharing their thoughts and personal experiences in working with this difficult patient population. They have been in the trenches. This book began with their concern for the recidivism of the symptoms and the light came on! This is addiction and, if not addressed, the danger is that the patients will switch to another and then another addiction. The book is filled with such stories. I knew Sandy and Cathy were good listeners.

*Sandra Steinbach, M.D., P.A.*

Psychiatry
1920 Abrams Parkway #376
Dallas, Texas 75214-3915

# A Note to the Reader

It might be that you have found a treatment situation in which you are encouraged to address all of your addictions and the ways that they interact, reinforce, and cover for each other. If that is the case, this book will be an excellent tool in your recovery. It will show you some of the ways that we and our patients have learned to track the connections among the powerful manifestations of the disease. If you are not in a situation in which you will receive simultaneous and integrated treatment, then this book will provide enormous benefit. Eventually, you will have to face up to and deal with the connections between your addictions and behaviors. If not, you may face a lifetime of relapses. Just as you gain traction in one area of your life, we believe that chances are you will slip and fall in another. This book is an invitation to you to start to think about the big picture, to start to think about how different forms of addictions and behaviors are attacking you at once. This book will guide you along the recovery road, physically, emotionally, mentally, socially, and most of all, spiritually.

During treatment, we recommend that patients with identified dual addictions or patients who would benefit from the education about dual addictions attend eating disorder sessions during the day and drug and alcohol sessions in the evening. We recommend the facilitation of weekly multifamily educational groups for parents, family members and others in the patients' support systems, and these sessions should be well attended by the patient's loved ones. We suggest that, in family group, the patients share the history, nature and extent of their eating disorders. We also encourage them to examine possible connections between their eating disorders and their histories of drug and alcohol use/abuse. From the moment of the first group meeting, we invite our patients to reflect upon and work toward their full recovery. As you will learn in later chapters, we sustain this integrated attention throughout the course of the patient's recovery.

We are convinced that addressing your eating disorders and chemical dependencies simultaneously can give you the healing power of full recovery.

## How to Read This Book

We suggest that you read in a way that you never have before: read these stories by writing your own. We ask you to purchase a writing notebook in order to journal and to create your story.

Your first step in your journey to recovery is to sign the front of the journal. Once you have done this, you have signed a contract with yourself. Your name is very important. Even if you feel like you don't know who you are right now, even if you feel that you have lost yourself, even if you hate yourself, or maybe you want to destroy yourself, your name is sacred. Your name is unique. Your name calls you into personhood. Sign this journal and even though you have written nothing else, you have started your journey.

You will write the following on the cover later.

TITLE

*(title)*

*The Story of My Simultaneous and Integrated Journey to Recovery*

BY

*(author)*

For now, leave the title blank. You will know when you are ready to give your recovery story a title. It might be when you are in the middle of your struggle with addiction that you most need a vision of something to work toward, a life that you want to achieve and accomplish. You might not be ready to title your journal until you have six months or one year to look back and reflect on your journey. You might have one word that sums up your experience and what you have learned. You might have a title that is much longer. You will know what to call your story when the time is right for you. For now, we just ask that you sign your name and that you keep up with the writing suggestions.

As you read, you will find a series of writing exercises that we ask you to complete. Clearly, unless you are reading this book with a treatment team or a therapist, no one is going to check on you and make sure that you are keeping up with your homework. However, you need to realize that to do your job you must write in your journal. Just reading, just waiting for us to fill your head with the knowledge that we have gained through our experience, is not enough. You must transform this knowledge into an awareness of your own recovery. That is why we ask that as you read, you create your own recovery story.

In the epilogue, you will find another invitation: We would like you to share the story of your integrated and simultaneous recovery journey with others. Our plan is to collect and publish the stories of women who are winning the war against dual addictions.

Chemical addictions and eating disorders reinforce and intensify a complicit and mutual devastation in the lives of countless women. Our patients already knew this. They knew that they became addicted to speed or cocaine to keep from eating; that they drank to keep from binging or to curb their appetite for food. They knew after purging that they were trying to drown their shame in bottles of vodka and gin. They knew that painkillers would numb the part of the brain that stimulates hunger. They also knew what happened when they kicked one of these addictions out the front door and tried to make their homes and their lives whole again. No sooner had they finished one treatment program, than the other behavior, the sinister complicit addiction, would slip in the back door and start the vicious cycle all over again.

We learned by observing these women that they had not just one addiction, but several addictions. We learned this while we were treating them. The recidivism rate of our patients was very high. Treatment became a swinging door and an operation for us to tackle both addictions at the same time. They came in for an eating disorder. They came back for a drug addiction. They left clean and sober. They came back starving. They came to us for binging. They came back drinking their lives away.

Eventually, we learned how to listen to our patients. We learned that they wanted help with their whole lives. They wanted freedom from both their raging chemical dependencies and the ravages of morbid and unhealthy eating disorders. These problems were ganging up on them, and they were tired of being treated for one, only to see the hidden addiction move in to overwhelm them.

So what's so revolutionary about this? The idea that programs should treat eating disorders and chemical dependencies in a simultaneous and integrated manner goes against a mountain of therapeutic orthodoxy. The received wisdom of the treatment community demands that patients address one addiction at a time. We shared this view. In fact, when we first met in a staff development meeting in 1998, we were hardly what you might call revolutionary voices. We were both part of the recovery establishment and we were both ready to fight for our own territory. Cathy had been hired as the new director of the chemical dependency unit at our medical center. Sandy had been the eating disorder program coordinator for many years. Our first conversation ran about 30 seconds and went something like this: "It will be fine, Cathy, to have your chemical dependency program here as long as your patients don't mingle with ours." "Don't worry, Sandy. Nobody is going to mingle."

After all these years of friendship, as we sit to write this book together, it is hard to believe that our first words to each other were both so cold and so close-minded. But we were typical of the treatment establishment. The lines between programs are distinct. Even today, many treatment programs send the same boxed-in message: Treatment programs will not mingle.

We have come a long way from that first meeting, in both our friendship and our thinking. We believe that women and men who face the dual or even multiple ordeals of chemical dependencies and eating disorders and concurrent psychiatric disorders need something different. Women facing these problems deserve more than counselors fighting to maintain their professional territory. When we decided to work together for the common good of the patient, we started seeing patients get well. Many women who treated the dual addictions were coming back to our aftercare program and testifying that they had been in recovery from their disease for two years. We learned that patients deserved a book, a resource that talks about problems with speed, cocaine and opiates to suppress appetite, drinking to help with purging or appetite suppression, because they want all of their life back, not just a part of it.

When women learn to face the voices of addiction and know that they are doing so, it is a powerful tool in their recovery and a giant leap toward a deeper understanding of themselves. The disease of addiction has learned how to twist this message. More and more often, we have seen the voices of these diseases agree to treat one addiction so that it can hide and nurture another:

"I only have one addiction, and anything else I do that seems like an addiction is not really a problem. I am in recovery, I wouldn't lie!"

"I can admit that I have an eating disorder. If I like to drink, that's no big deal. If it ever becomes a big deal, I will treat it later. Smoking pot daily isn't a big deal. After all, pot isn't really a drug."

"I have come a long way, and I know I am anorexic. I only use cocaine and meth when I party with my friends, it's social. It's not like the two are related."

When our patients talk to us like this, they are in denial. They are using their recovery from one addiction to camouflage and protect the growth of another addiction or destructive behavior. This is recovery double-talk. These are the women who come back again and again to treatment programs. They shop around and blame their lack of success on the facility, the doctors and the counselors. These women make progress with one addiction only to find their lives spinning out of control in another area. These women enter an eating disorder unit and are released. A year later, they enter a chemical dependency unit for behavior that used to be "no big deal." These are women with dual or multiple addictions, right along with major depression or the other disorders being in the mix of it all.

We believe that these women need to face their addictions and behaviors in an integrated and simultaneous treatment program because the addictions certainly attack them simultaneously. We have learned that behaviors reinforce each other and that treating one addiction while ignoring another can lead to catastrophe. We predict that in the future many therapists and treatment facilities will choose to integrate their eating disorder and chemical dependency protocol.

We also have come to appreciate the suffering the families always face when they have a loved one who is battling these devastating diseases. This book will be a great resource for you, the family or anyone who has a loved one battling an eating disorder or substance abuse problem. You will find hope and comfort from this chapter and learn how to not allow the disease to become a toxic waste dump in your soul, mind and body.

OPERATION *Daughters* ADDICTED

ONE

# Getting To Know You: The First Step Toward Full Recovery

*You know who* you are.

You're walking down the aisle of the grocery store and saying, "If I could, I would sample every piece of food. I'll buy my binge food, take it home, pull the blinds and get into my comfortable hiding place and eat, and eat and eat. When I'm through, I'll throw it up. I'll open a bottle of wine in order to feel better and escape the madness of my behavior."

"I'm the young woman who likes to wear size one and size two clothing and I know that I can't have a morsel of food in order to accomplish this goal. I'm the woman who loves to cook for everyone, but won't allow myself to taste one bite of food. I drink Chinese herbal tea in order to curb my appetite. I use methamphetamine or cocaine to keep the hunger pangs from gnawing at me."

"I'm the woman who is large and hides behind the food and alcohol in order to soothe my pain. I drive to different fast food restaurants to feed my food addiction. The car looks like a trash bin. But I can't allow anyone to know just how much I really eat. I can look at a loaf of bread in the grocery store and count how many sandwiches that the loaf make. My shame is great and wrapped in a big meal."

Now, we want to know you.

There's an old song written by Oscar and Hammerstein and sung by Julie Andrews with a hook that goes, "Getting to know you." We wanted to start with this song from *The King and I* because it puts to music our first theme: Getting to know you. It might seem strange that from the first page in a book about the combined oppressions of chemical addictions and eating disorders, we are talking about getting to know you instead of you discovering the lessons we have to offer. But the song puts it all in perspective. In the movie, Andrews plays a teacher who has been chosen to educate the king's children. She learns very quickly, like many teachers, that in reality she is the one who stands to learn the most from her students. The song reveals an important lesson that we have learned in our combined 67 years of clinical experience in treating eating disorders and chemical dependency at noted psychiatric facilities. We learned the most about these diseases when we learned how to listen to our patients. Our patients made the strongest recoveries when they learned how to listen to themselves.

We are offering you a unique opportunity on your road to recovery. We want to get to know you. We want you to get to know yourself. We want you to get to know us. If you were in the dual-addiction program at our hospital, we would remain anonymous so that the focus remained entirely on you and the other patients making the recovery journey with you. In writing this book, we want to offer something different. We want to take the recovery journey with you. You see, we too have struggled with the diseases of addiction and eating disorders. We want to share our struggles with you to let you know that you are not alone.

We also want to remind you that we are real people. People trapped by addictions and obsessed by negative body image and eating habits forget to look at themselves and others as real people. We understand the voices of concurrent addictions and how they aid and abet each other. The committee voices in your head tell you ongoing lies. Drugs and alcohol are always at the door knocking and, if you open the door, they have you. If you start to binge, the voices in your head lie and tell you to get rid of the calories by vomiting and to drink alcohol because it will make it easier to purge. For the overeater, alcohol will enable you to drink and eat less. Pain pills will allow you to kill the pangs of hunger. The addiction voice will tell you to do meth and you won't have to eat today. For the addict, for the anorexic, for the bulimic, people are nothing more than cogs in the addiction wheel: Who can get me my drugs? Who can tell me it's okay to binge and purge because I just broke up with my boyfriend or separated from my husband? Who will stay out late and party with me, even though I have commitments the next morning?

In very subtle ways, addicts know who will enable their diseases and who will try to confront them about their behaviors. They use all of their skills to practice their eating disorder. They are often very gifted women who use their gifts to deceive themselves and those around them: From whom do I need to hide my addictions? Who will confront me openly and honestly about what I am doing to myself? Who refuses to look the other way? When addicts think like this, they are avoiding people. They are speaking the language of the disease. They are even ignoring themselves by only listening to the voice of their addictions.

There are many excellent books on the market that can help people recover from all kinds of addictions and behaviors. This book will probably not be the only one you read on your journey. It shouldn't be. You are going to come across great books in the recovery field. Some will be recommended by friends and family, your therapist and counselors will lead you to some and some you will find on your own. We believe that our book offers a unique perspective. Most books that tackle problems with chemical dependency and eating disorders ask you to confront one addiction at a time. This one-addiction-at-a-time method is part of a long-standing treatment philosophy in the field. But we know how important it is to eliminate all addictions, given our own battles to become healthy and we wish this treatment philosophy for all the millions of women who struggle with addictions.

When a patient says that she is willing to choose the recovery journey, it is an empowering moment. She has started to respond, according to the Alcoholics Anonymous Big Book, to a disease that is "cunning, baffling and powerful" and that constantly undermines her judgment, self-esteem, and self-control by bombarding her with all-or-nothing scenarios. The voices of the disease say: If you are not the best at your job, you are worthless. You may as well use your drug of choice. You can control your drinking this time and only have one beer.

Before going any further in this book, we would like to take a brief account of who we are. You see the problems of addiction and eating disorders are not just professional concerns. They have also deeply affected our personal lives.

## Cathy

"Hi, my name is Cathy. I'm an alcoholic." Introductions like this are heard every day in Alcoholics Anonymous meetings around the world. I could have saved myself 15 years of misery if knowledge about the genetic basis of alcoholism had been as advanced then as it is today. I now know that I'm loaded genetically with the predisposition for alcoholism, and I know that I'm an alcoholic. My father was a recovering alcoholic. My brother died of liver failure due to alcoholism. I have a number of other close family members who have died as a result of addiction. I took my first drink at 16 and never really stopped until I entered substance abuse treatment 16 years later, in 1978. My struggle for sobriety echoes throughout this book. Getting sober was difficult, but not as difficult as trying to live in this world without a buffer like alcohol. I knew that I needed to replace this disease with something constructive, so I worked the 12 Steps and continue to work number 12 to this day (please see the 12 Steps on page 174.)

I am a counselor and have never once thought about any profession other than working with patients facing alcoholism and addictions. I have seen the devastation that this disease can cause. I am still amazed that in many families where lives are destroyed by alcoholism or drug addiction, even with all the information we have learned in the last 30 years, alcoholism remains the "elephant in the living room." I have seen addicts who have lost everything and end up homeless because of their heroin or cocaine addiction. I have seen children farmed out to strangers because their once beautiful mother could no longer take care of them. I have seen the diseases of addiction take down powerful men who were chief executive officers of major corporations. I have seen NFL players sit permanently on the sideline because of their cocaine habit. Actors, actresses and models have passed by my counseling couch. I have heard them tell the same sad story of how it started with the partying, but the party never stopped. The daily encounters with other alcoholics and addicts has been a blessing in my life, because with each counseling session or each consult I realized that there go I, but by the grace of God. For my complete story, turn to chapter five.

## Sandy

My name is Sandy, and I want to tell you my story. After completing a nursing degree in the late 1960s, I worked in Cleveland for five years. I then became a Peace Corps volunteer in Iran, where I met my husband who was also a volunteer. I stayed at home for 14 years raising our three sons. During a nursing refresher course, I decided to return to the profession working as a nurse in psychiatry. To enhance my diploma, I also went back to school to become a licensed chemical dependency counselor. Little did I realize how these simple choices would change my life by working with women facing the trauma of eating disorders became my professional passion. I have worked with the eating disorder programs of two nationally renowned medical centers for more than 20 years.

Working with these women also opened my eyes to my own compulsive overeating and my personal 12 Step recovery journey. In my family of origin, I can trace four generations of women with eating disorders, including anorexia nervosa, bulimia nervosa and binge eating. My mother's family had always been obsessed with physical beauty. The family ideal was painfully typical: tall with blond hair and blue eyes and most importantly, rail thin. I never measured up. Today, I am still short with green eyes. I do have blond hair, thanks to my hair stylist. The greatest tragedy, from the warped perspective I inherited from a nutritionally dysfunctional family, is that I am overweight. To this day, and despite my continual admonitions, when my mother sees someone from my past, she begins our conversation by telling me how much he or she weighs.

Alcoholism flows freely on both sides of my family. My biological father, with whom I was not raised, died drunk. My favorite aunt was an alcoholic. I have a brother who is alcoholic, and my husband's father was alcoholic. I bring these memories to work with me every day. I know that the devastation wreaked by the disease of addiction doesn't just happen to other people and other people's families. This devastation touches all of us. For my complete story, turn to chapter six.

## Your Personal Story

It is now time to start writing your story in your journal. At the end of each chapter, we will include a scripture passage to meditate upon, or you may prefer using the meaningful quote as your meditation theme. Below you will find the first meditation and instruction on how to meditate. You will use the same meditation method throughout the book. The commentary is a guide to help you soul search while pondering the answer to the questions that we have provided. Please use this commentary to guide you into your journey of getting to know yourself. Throughout the book, you will find questions to answer and a commentary on how to get started with meditation at the end of each chapter. This process is an exciting time for you and your recovery.

# Assignment for Chapter One

## PSALM 25:4

Your ways, Oh God, make known to me;
Teach me your paths.
The living and true God directs
Our coming and going.

## Quote

In the next century
Or the one beyond that
They say,
Are valleys, pastures.

We can meet there in peace
If we make it.
To climb these coming crests
One word to you, to
You and your children:

Stay together
Learn the flowers
Go light.

Gary Snyder, Name of Poem: unnamed. This was taken out of the book *Prayers for a Thousand Years* edited by Elizabeth Roberts & Elias Amidon, publisher Harper San Francisco, copyright 1999.

## Meditation Exercise

1. Find a quiet place. Focus and center your attention to your breathing. Let go of your thoughts and worries. Then, slowly say the poem or verse (Psalm 25:4) as you direct your attention to God or your higher power.
2. Repeat the verse a number of times. Digest the poem or verse, for this is truly soul food.
3. Reflect on what the poem or verse is saying to you at this moment. What do you need to let go of or change in order to follow God's or your higher power's path, to follow His way for you? When you complete the work of this meditation, express gratitude for what you have learned and determine in some simple way how you will honor the gift that has come to you from this meditation

## Commentary

Sometimes it amazes us. We turn to the Scriptures, seeking food for the soul, and a verse leaps out at us and pierces the heart. We are touched by the right words at the right moment. Psalm 25:4 has taken on a very special meaning for us. We always want to do it our way. That's what we've done all our lives. No one can tell us anything. On the outside, we do our best to look good, but the truth is that we can't keep it all together anymore. Our lives are a mess. They're full of lies and deceit. We end up pushing away the people we love and care about. That's why this verse is so striking. We are not alone in this thing called life. I really don't stand by myself as if it's me against the world. We are part of something so much greater than ourselves. For the first time in our lives, we are really ready to listen: to acknowledge you, oh God, and from the depths of our being implore you to make known to us your ways and to show us your paths.

## Questions

1. What is my first recollection of an eating disorder? Give a detailed example and write a timeline of usage throughout your life up to present. Think hard and don't leave anything out. For example, do you remember the first day you decided you wouldn't eat for the entire day? How soon after that day did you repeat the pattern? Do you remember the first time you felt full and decided it would be better to get rid of the food instead of feeling uncomfortable?
2. When did I first use a mood altering substance, alcohol, speed, coke, pain pills, or marijuana? Give a detailed example and write a time line of usage throughout your life.
3. Does my timeline reveal my actual eating disorder and chemical use history accurately?
4. Does my disease history show a correlation between the eating disorder and the chemical usage? Does it appear to me that I've used chemicals to help me maintain my eating disorder?

TWO

# Preparing for the Big Picture Intake: Your Life in the Mirror

CHAPTER OBJECTIVES

✓ *See how addictions destroy your physical health*

✓ *See the stronghold of denial*

✓ *See the "big picture."*

*In this chapter,* we invite you to complete what we call the big picture intake of mind, body, and spirit. During the big picture intake, you will declare your baggage as you take the first step on your journey of recovery. We will ask you to look at the state of your life and your health, honestly and openly. We will invite you to make an inventory of your whole life: eating habits, sleeping patterns, physical activities and physical health. We will also ask you to contemplate the health of your soul and your quest for spirituality. Don't underestimate the importance of taking in this big picture. Once you realize where you are, then you will be able to decide where you want to go and how you want to get there.

Okay, this sounds simple. But we have learned from hundreds of patients that honestly assessing their own big picture is one of the most difficult parts of the journey. In fact, right now, you might not even be able to admit to yourself that you have an eating disorder, let alone a chemical dependency problem, not even to yourself. Just think, if you can't admit that you are starving yourself to death, that you aren't just throwing up a big lunch but rather throwing away your life, that you are toasting your own death every time you open another bottle of wine or vodka, then how can you imagine talking about it? How can you imagine talking to other people with the same problems? How can you imagine telling a therapist, "I have an eating disorder and a problem with alcohol, and I am killing myself." Worst of all, how can you imagine getting better?

These questions paint a dramatic picture, and they must. A saying in the treatment community about the life-or-death choice that people with eating disorders and chemical addictions face is, there are only two ways out of an addiction: recovery or death. You choose.

Don't assume that the choice is either easy or obvious. We see people make the wrong choice every day. Working with patients battling alcoholism, chemical addictions, and eating disorders has taught us that the disease of addiction is a killer. We both have seen this again and again. We both have stories to share.

## Two Patients and Two Big Pictures

### JESSE

As you now know, I, Cathy, am a recovering alcoholic and professional counselor. Fighting this disease has been a continual learning and growing experience for me. The violence and confusion of addictions still astound me. I remember an alcoholism consultation for a patient in the medical unit of our hospital late one cold winter evening. My first inclination was to put it off until the next day. Instead, I grudgingly left the psychiatry building, made the trek across to the main hospital and took the elevator to the seventh floor. Entering the room, I encountered Jesse, a handsome man, about 40 years old, scowling at me from a hospital bed. His stomach was distended. It looked like a basketball under his hospital robe. Clearly, I was dealing with someone who was in the beginning stages of liver failure. His body was starting to collapse from the onslaught of the disease. I could see his life sinking in the yellow haze of his eyes. My first job was to diagnose his alcoholism:

"When did you start drinking?"

"I was around fourteen years old. Everybody in my family drank. My daddy died because of it."

"How much do you drink now?"

"Eighteen to twenty beers a day."

"Is there alcoholism in your family?"

"My two brothers, my daddy and all his brothers."

"Are there job and family problems?"

"Some." He didn't elaborate. Instead, he looked at his wife and young son who were still in the room.

Finally, I asked, "Do you have physical problems as a result of your drinking?" Everyone who had come to the hospital room that night knew the answer. Jesse, his stomach distended, his skin yellow, his body smelling like it was rotting from the inside out, was a full-blown alcoholic. Despite the clarity of the situation, when I told him that he needed to go for long-term treatment for alcoholism, he responded angrily, "I need to get the hell out of here, that's what I need." Seeing his five-year-old son at his bedside, I chose my words carefully. "Unless you go for long-term treatment and learn how not to drink, you will not get well." He and his wife started to argue at this point. I excused myself and went into the hallway to document my findings in his medical chart.

I looked up over my glasses. From around the corner, his son was watching me. "What's going to happen to my daddy?" I was caught off guard and said very quickly, "Your daddy is going to be your daddy." His wife came rushing out of the room, grabbed the young boy's hand and took off down the corridor. I re-entered Jesse's room, stood at the foot of the bed, and for a split second I saw myself lying in that bed 23 years before. I, too, was helpless, sick and terrified. I thought I would never be able to let go of my disease. I asked Jesse to reconsider going for long-term treatment. I went around to the side of his bed and knelt down just inches away from his face. I whispered, "If you don't do this for yourself, then do it for that little boy." The man began to cry. I saw at that moment that he was finally taking in the big picture. That night, I watched God move in both of our lives. It took the power of God to help him realize that he was killing himself and his family. God helped him take his first step toward health and happiness. At that time, God reminded me that I'm only His instrument, a messenger to carry the gifts of His love and power.

The next morning, the nurse from the unit called me to tell me Jesse had decided to go for long-term alcohol treatment.

Two years later, Jesse came up to the psych unit to visit me. He had his young son with him. I barely recognized Jesse due to his now healthy, less-emaciated frame. He began to tell me how life had changed for him and his family: "I've kept the same job now for two years. Me and my wife are expecting another child."

I held back tears as I praised his successful recovery, "Jesse, are you going to AA?"

"Yes, and better than that," he said, "I'm attending church."

I asked him, "What really clicked for you?"

"My boy," he said. "I wanted things to be different for him. You know, break the cycle, like you said."

### APRIL

I, Sandy, have been astounded by the disease's power of denial. At times, I do intake evaluations for admission into an eating disorder program. The number of women who defend their diseases, even as the diseases ravage them, devastates me. Frequently, patients have injured their health so severely that they are rushed to the emergency room and end up being admitted to the cardiac unit to be stabilized medically before they can be admitted to the eating disorder unit.

Several years ago, I made a trip to the hospital's cardiac unit to evaluate a patient for the eating disorder program. Because the evaluation took place in April, I will call the patient April. I walked into her room and saw a bedridden, frail figure being kept alive by a feeding tube, an IV, a catheter and heart monitoring equipment. Most of her hair was gone. She was covered with sores. Her body and hollowed-out face told the whole story: She was dying. April was in her early 40s, and, at five-feet-four-inches tall, she weighed barely 60 pounds. One of the remaining signs of life was her deep blue eyes. But even these were not vigorous, hopeful or fighting for the future. They had been taken over by the forces of the disease. They darted suspiciously from me to the body over whose demise they were keeping cruel vigilance.

April had come from California to seek treatment because she heard that we were part of a medical center that could address her severe medical complications. She claimed to be allergic to most foods. She had been living only on select vegetables for the last several months. She had collapsed from worsening malnutrition and had been rushed to the hospital a number of times in her hometown. Her trip to our treatment program literally could have been one of her last.

She was desperate. April was fighting for her life. To my amazement, however, she was also fighting to kill herself. Even in her compromised medical condition, April's first words to me showed that she was willing to risk everything to practice her eating disorder:

"You don't understand. I really am allergic to food."

"My other doctors told me I can eat what I am comfortable with."

"I am thin because my whole family is thin."

"I just have a weak heart, and that is why I am here."

"Let me work my way back to larger meals."

"I am sick right now. I don't feel like eating."

"I don't want to gain all that weight back."

"I'll get fat if I eat again. I'm big boned."

April was willing to let this cruel addiction take her life. She was even willing to aid and abet the disease.

Part of our job as counselors is to speak the truth to the manipulating powers of the disease. Because of this, I strive to be matter-of-fact with information about the program, and I resist escalating melodramatic scenes. In this spirit, I assured April that our dietitians would assign a regimen of therapeutic meals and snacks. She would be required to consume a prescribed number of calories and portions. She would not be able to exercise food restrictions. Any alleged allergies were to be confirmed through a medical diagnosis. To take part in our program meant that April would have to agree to eat all food placed before her. She would also have to submit to drug and alcohol screenings and, for the foreseeable future, she would have to refrain from exercise. I believe that the best service for new patients coming into an eating disorder program is not to have any surprises about the program and philosophy of treatment. These guidelines ask the patients to care for the fundamentals of their physical health. Essentially, the guidelines say, "Eat and live."

At first, April would have none of it. Those steel-blue eyes were not giving up without a fight. Not until two more weeks in critical condition, both physically and spiritually, did she consent to the program guidelines. It took her entire family, and I believe the power of God, to give April the strength to realize that she was killing herself and sacrificing the mental health of her family as well. It still overwhelms me that April was pushed to her deathbed before she agreed to take in her big picture.

April came into the program and did a complete course of treatment. Her husband and her parents also came to the unit and did family work. Because April was so physically compromised, she was an inpatient for almost two months. She then transitioned to day hospital treatment, where she stayed in the hotel on campus at night. When she was an inpatient, her weight gain was reasonable, that is, around two pounds a week. As soon as April was in day hospital, her weight gain slowed and came to a halt within a couple of weeks. She was able to gain weight when under 24-hour supervision as a hospital inpatient. Sadly, as a day hospital patient left to her own devices in the evening, she was exercising calories away. At the time of discharge, she smiled and promised to follow her meal plan and not exercise when she went home until her heart was healthy again. April has not contacted the program since she was discharged. Many of our patients come to the aftercare group when they are in town or they call or send pictures to tell us that they are in recovery, they just want to touch base with us again. I wonder how April's life is going and fear the worst. I wonder if she isn't playing the deadly game with her eating disorder, living on the fence between life and death and holding those who love her hostage.

## The Courage to Face the Physical Damage

As you start to examine your own big picture, we first ask that you acknowledge the physical damage that has occurred from practicing your eating disorder and/or abusing drugs and/or alcohol. If we were able to treat you in person, we would ask you to submit to a complete medical workup, including an echo-cardiogram, a bone density scan, blood tests and drug and alcohol screenings. These tests help us lay the groundwork for recovery. They identify heart damage and bone loss due to malnutrition. They paint an honest picture of your fitness and physical strength. Furthermore, they begin to explain how the use of chemical substances has enabled the eating disorder. Complications associated with eating disorders and substance abuse are varied and extreme.

The physical damage that occurs when someone practices an eating disorder and chemical addiction includes muscle loss, which occurs from malnutrition. The body does everything possible to survive. The body uses fat reserves and then starts to eat muscle. Because the heart is a muscle, at some point in the starvation process, the body starts to cannibalize the heart, which may result in thinning of the heart wall, leaking heart valves, enlargement of the aortic root, fluid around the heart and enlargement of a heart chamber. Heart damage may also be brought on by the force of repeated vomiting.

The valves of the heart may become damaged from repeated vomiting, abuse of laxatives, starvation and dehydration, which cause a life-threatening situation. Heartburn, stomach pain, sore throat and constipation are symptoms of repeated vomiting and starvation. Osteoporosis (bone loss) is caused by lack of adequate vitamins and calcium in the diet. Loss of menstrual period may also affect bones and the potential for fertility. Sexual drive will most likely be decreased or non-existent. For many others, the sex drive may be affected so severely that they resort to using cocaine or methamphetamine, which often happens. These drugs only give them a false sense of a heightened sex drive. In addition to the above, because of increased vomiting, the enamel of the teeth gets worn away, exposing the teeth to decay. Starvation also negatively affects teeth and gums.

When alcohol is put into the mix with the eating disorder, liver disease (cirrhosis) is prevalent. The heart can become enlarged. Heavy consumption of alcohol is thought to cause enlargement through three mechanisms: (1) a direct toxic effect of alcohol or of its metabolites; (2) effects of nutritional deficits, especially thiamine deficiency; (3) toxic effects of beverage additives such as cobalt. Cocaine and methamphetamine will cause the depletion of a neurotransmitter, dopamine. Dopamine is one of the "feel good" chemicals in the brain and is responsible for learning, attention and emotion. Cocaine and methamphetamine can cause a heart attack, especially in an anorexic because the heart is already compromised due to the lack of proper nutrition. The list of physical damage from the two diseases goes on and on.

Lesley Williams M.D., an internist for the treatment facility, Remuda Ranch, located in Wickenburg, Arizona, gave us the opportunity to interview her regarding some of the newest findings in women who have been active in their disease for years. Dr. William's assessment of young women and the physical damage she is seeing in her patients at Remuda Ranch are through the CAT SCAN image of the brain.Dr. Williams said the most worrisome physical damage is to the brain. The scans are showing brain shrinkage due to years of starvation. Young, bright women who have practiced their disordered eating for a number of years are now unable to function due to their inability to hold or maintain memory.

We've worked with many intelligent and caring professionals in our professional journey. One in particular who has done some extensive research in the area of Eating Disorders is Dr. Jim Harris a Clinical Psychologist and Clinical Director of the Eating Disorder program at Presbyterian Hospital of Dallas. Dr. Harris states that recent advances in neuroscience are catching up to what we've known through clinical wisdom. For example, functional magnetic resonance imaging (fMRI) provides a moving picture of brain functions. Researchers were startled to discover that self-identity in people suffering from anorexia was less developed than those who had schizophrenia or Asperger's disease. Clinical wisdom has informed that one of the most difficult tasks is helping patients separate themselves form their eating disorder, process of developing identity. The findings from fMRI research now confirm why this task is so challenging.

Treatment implications include re-focusing on interpersonal therapy as a means of helping develop identify. Development psychology informs that identity is developed in part through relationships with significant others. Techniques fostering such may be emphasized over more traditional cognitive behavioral approaches.

Neuropsychological findings also confirm clinical wisdom. For example, those suffering from anorexia are found to have significant difficulty with se-shifting. This means that in problem solving they tend to cling to familiar patterns rather than attempt novel problem solutions. For those suffering with bulimia marked problems with impulse control are noted. Findings suggest interconnections vital to problem solving, understanding consequences, self-identity and delaying gratification, does not fully become operational until age 25. Guess what happens if one adds malnutrition, drugs or alcohol to the developing brain? While this research remains to be done, it does not seem a stretch to imagine that brain development would slow down. Treatment implications include continued focus on nutritional rehabilitation and abstinence from alcohol and drugs.

## Praying for your Big Picture

Once you begin to take stock of the physical damage that the eating disorder is inflicting upon your body, we suggest you turn inward and assess the state of your soul.

In this final section of the intake chapter, we provide spiritual meditations to help prepare for the big picture. Reading this book is a great spiritual, intellectual and physical challenge. By the end of this journey, you will be ready to face the fact that by practicing your eating disorder and chemical/alcohol dependency, you are participating in your own destruction. In effect, you are killing yourself, slowly but surely.

## Assignment for Chapter Two

### PSALM 25:9

He guides the humble to justice.
He teaches the humble His way.

## Quote

Something was dead in each of us,
And what was dead was Hope.

Oscar Wilde, The Ballad of Reading Gaol, III, St. 3

### Meditate and reflect on the psalm or quote

## Commentary

As we mentioned at the end of chapter One, we have selected some of our favorite psalms and inspirational quotes for you to contemplate. You might have read these beautiful prayers and quotes before. We ask you this time to turn to them to ask yourself and God for the guidance to take in the big picture of your disease. Use these psalms and quotes courageously and honestly to assess your physical, mental and spiritual health. We will provide commentaries and questions to guide your journey of discovery.

There is an ancient monastic meditation practice called *lectio divina*. *Lectio divina*, soul food. Begin by choosing a brief passage of Scripture. We attentively read the words and may repeat phrases. With our imaginations, we picture ourselves in the scene. With each of our senses, we appropriate, we enhance our image of the scene. With the mind, we seek to understand the meaning of the passage. With our hearts, we receive the words of the Scripture or beautiful quote into ourselves. We take the words into our hearts for nourishment and, through meditation, our lives become transformed.

The journey we take is unique, but each journey requires us to be willing, humble and receptive. It's so easy to let time pass without taking responsibility for ourselves, without taking ownership of our own part of any of our relationships. Psalm 25:9 expresses a humble request for Divine guidance in our lives. God knows how slow we are to learn what we need to know, even though it's so simple to learn to follow His path. If we had a nickel for every time we've seen the Word humble in the Scriptures, we'd be rich. The question is: What does it mean to be humble? Somehow, the word has taken on a connotation of being wimpy. In Scripture, however, humble refers accepting the truth of ourselves. It's the ability to see ourselves as we really are and to see ourselves in relationship to all beings, to the earth, and to the Divine. Why is this so hard for us? Why do we grasp at so many phony things? We know, at least in rare moments of truth about ourselves, that our addictions feed the illusions we have.

## Questions to Answer

1. List the ways that you have damaged your body by practicing your eating disorder and/or your drug and alcohol use/abuse.
2. Write about your relationship with your family, friends, and significant others. How have your relationships been damaged? Be specific.
3. Write about your emotional health. Are you able to feel feelings, or are you numbed out? Is anger the only feeling you are able to express?
4. Write about your spiritual life. What do you believe in spiritually?
5. What do you need to let go of to be humble?
6. Are you willing to take this journey with yourself? If so then you're ready to move to number 7.
7. List goals that will enhance your physical, mental, emotional, social and spiritual health. This may even have you changing some friendships.

THREE

# Tapestries of Life: Real Stories from Real People

**CHAPTER OBJECTIVES**

✓ *Show how we came to understand the connections among multiple addictions.*

✓ *Show how the patients came to realize their addictions were interconnected.*

✓ *Invite you to explore the negative connections among your addictions.*

We would now like to share composites of real stories from real people. In the profession, these are known as "case histories." To our ears, this term sounds too clinical. After all, these patients' struggles aren't just statistics or experiments. These are true-to-life stories that opened our eyes to how chemical and alcohol addictions act together with eating disorders to destroy women's lives. The life-changing stories are the flesh and blood of this book. The women who spent so much time destroying their own bodies have given life to the body of this book and by extension will reinvigorate the bodies and souls of our readers. What a miracle of the recovery process!

However, from the beginning, we struggled with how to present these stories to our readers. These patients told powerful tales of overcoming addiction. We learned from them every day as we sat across from them in private counseling sessions, next to them in group therapy and with them at the dinner table. But short of inviting you into our offices, into our group sessions or to our table, how could we convey these powerful lessons to you? Ultimately, we came to an epiphany: Yes, these women were amazing teachers, but there was more to the story. We were gifted learners, and we had gained a unique knowledge: We had been blessed with the ability to see connections.

We were able to make what the Greek philosophers first called a *diagnosis* (the Greek term is *dia*); through these stories, we gained knowledge (the Greek term is *gnosis*) of the disease and their symptoms. We grasped the big picture that lay beyond the chaos wreaking havoc in these women's lives. Listening to how eating disorders and chemical and alcohol abuse tightened their stranglehold over countless women, we witnessed larger patterns emerge. We saw again and again how these dual addictions aided and abetted each other. We observed hundreds of women seeking treatment for one condition only to have a complicit disorder intensify and undo any advances made.

Once we understood that we had gained a special wisdom from our work, we came to a second realization: We could share our newfound understanding with others. So we embraced the ancient practice of storytelling, the practice that has long been the domain of healers. In almost all cultures, women have a special relationship to recounting and listening to stories. We began to rediscover the power of storytelling all around us. In our own lives as we thought back to our childhoods and our earliest memories, it was our mothers, grandmothers, aunts and sisters who imparted to us our earliest wisdom.

Understanding the power of storytelling clarified our mission in writing this book. Our job is to use our own creative powers to weave the individual threads of these patients' lives into a vital and vibrant tapestry for our readers. The best way to share these stories is to allow our creative powers to do their part. Our creativity can condense and fashion these tales, combine the manifold isolated truths into the big picture truth. From shredded lives, we have woven a whole and healing tapestry.

When you read the stories in this chapter, you may have a straightforward reaction. You are going to think, "These stories are real. I know they're real because the same thing happened to me." You are absolutely right. These stories are real because we have made up nothing. We have taken true experiences from several patients in order to provide you with composite case histories of patients who we have named Amanda, Heather and Kerry. These are the hard and fast facts experienced by countless women whom we have counseled.

Eating disorders, drinking and taking drugs will destroy women's natural powers of creation and creativity. Countless times we have seen our patients learn and share this lesson. In a group session, we heard one patient tell another, "But look at what you just said. You told us that your dream has always been to make a family, and yet you are destroying the same part of you that will make that family. You are destroying your womb!" We have heard gifted athletes say they can no longer climb a flight of stairs. We have heard college students struggle with subtracting 7 from 100. We have heard women tell us that they could not even imagine what a better life would be like. Their powers to imagine, live and create were so compromised they could not even envision what getting better would be like.

In response to this destruction of creation and creativity, we have used our creative power to tell stories. We also want you to use your creative powers. Nature has given women the power to create, to give birth, to imagine and transform. This power can help you counteract and defeat the diseases devastating you.

You can use your creative powers in two ways. First, be an imaginative reader. As you read these stories, we want you to use your imagination to place yourself beside them. Envision how they parallel your life; consider the details that echo with what has happened to you. Don't just see your life in the misery of these voices. Identify with the victories.

Awaken your creative power and become a part of the recovering community.

Second, be a creative writer. We want you to go a step further than merely imagining how these stories relate to you. It may sound strange, but don't just read these stories. Write them. The assignments at the end of each chapter are very important. Only by exploring the connections between eating disorders and alcoholism and drug addiction in your own words and in your own life will you come to a true revelation of your particular situation.

This chapter will present the stories of three eating disorder patients who struggled for years with anorexia, bulimia, binge eating, purging and starvation. Through the course of their recovery, we discovered, with help from these remarkable patients, that they also suffered from years of covert drug addiction and alcohol abuse.

Looking back, we wonder how we could have missed it. These women were bent on hiding their eating disorders but at times were strangely open with their descriptions of drug and alcohol use. According to the messed-up logic of these concurrent diseases, drinking and drugging "was not a problem" for them and there was therefore "nothing to hide." They even admitted to using drugs and alcohol "occasionally" or "socially" or maybe only "when my friends were doing it." Initially, we missed how these furtive behaviors were aiding and abetting their eating disorders. Instead, as the profession had trained us, we paid little attention to the alcohol and drug use and focused on the eating disorders.

This chapter presents stories of patients who we first met in our chemical dependency and alcohol abuse programs. Peeling back the layers of pain and devastation that shrouded their lives, we discovered self-hatred had propelled them into the destruction of their bodies through eating disorders. Alcohol and drug use furthered the destruction. Our training had taught us to identify and treat these conditions separately, so the revelation of their interconnection was a major paradigm shift. Our main goal in these chapters is to help you make a similar revelation in your own life. Once the interconnections among your conditions have been revealed, you can proceed to a whole recovery with full awareness.

The message from both of these chapters should be as clear to you as it was to us. Women deserve more than arbitrary and isolated treatment for their conditions. Women deserve, you deserve, simultaneous and integrated treatment for eating disorders and alcohol/drug dependencies, simultaneous and integrated treatment that heals whole lives.

## Three Patients, Three Stories

Kerry was an especially troubled adolescent who we treated in the eating disorder program. She had struggled as a teen to overcome a drinking problem. When we met her, she had just started to work through the shame and devastation of being molested by a neighbor. Kerry was withdrawn, cautious, intelligent and not in touch with her feelings. We want to share her story first because for us she represents all the hope of youth facing problems but unable to overcome these problems. When we met her, she was not able to overcome them because she was not able to face her big picture. Kerry is not just an alcoholic. She is also a drug addict with a severe eating disorder.

We want you to listen to Kerry's initial reaction to visiting our eating disorder program. Days earlier, she had been admitted to the cardiac unit for the beginning signs of heart failure, an immediate effect of years of self-enforced starvation. Despite the threatening severity of her condition, she agreed to enter the eating disorder program only "to make her parents happy." As you read, notice how Kerry has to fight the forces of two potentially fatal disorders to ask for the help that she so desperately, and obviously, needs.

### KERRY

So, they want me to reflect back on my initial tour of their eating disorder program and my decision to enter treatment? OK.

Well, to start, I remember that the tour was an ordeal. Talk about wanting to scream. I didn't want to be locked up like a rat. Did freedom mean nothing to these people? I mean, I was already locked up for two weeks getting sober. Now they wanted me to be locked up because they claim I'm anorexic?

That was something that always bothered me: all the diagnoses they made as if they really knew what was going on. I didn't believe that my heart was that bad. Permanent damage? Heart failure? I can't even exercise? Bed rest? Whatever! That doctor is just trying to scare me.

It really wasn't the doctors or the counselors who first got me to think about doing the program. It was the other patients. I remember what I said when I walked in the door: "Hi, I'm Kerry. I'm here to see the place to get my parents off my back. I don't really want to be here. I'm a vegetarian, not an anorexic! It's not like I need to be here."

But then that nurse Sandy started to confront me with the so-called "facts." The doctor had told her about my weak heart that had ended me up on the medical floor. Even though I knew it was true, I still hadn't put it together that I had dropped out of college because my weak heart was making me sick and I could no longer even think. But there it was, I had dropped out, and my doctor had spilled the beans to my parents, the echo-cardiogram results. Even though I had secretly known all along, hearing the damage from this nurse sort of stunned me. Next, she introduced some of the other patients in the program. She walked away saying, "I will be back in a few minutes. Ask all the questions on your mind." I know it sounds weird, but I can still remember those introductions:

"I'm Nancy. I'm anorexic-bulimic. I have been in the program for three weeks. I understand that you're feeling pressured about coming into the program. Well, I had a lot of pressure to come to treatment, too. My work insisted I get help and I didn't want to lose my job. My husband even said that our marriage was probably over if I didn't get some help."

"Hi Kerry, I'm Brittany, bulimic. I haven't purged in six weeks. That is the longest I have gone in four years.

"Hi Kerry, I'm Lisa. I was a vegetarian for eight years before I started the program. I took the same stance as you. After some soul searching, I decided that my life was too valuable and I was too close to death's door to argue. For me, being a vegetarian was too much a part of my eating disorder. I had only started out to eat healthily, and I ended up eliminating first the meat group, then the fat group, and then the carb group. This is where it got me."

"I'm Melissa. The locked doors terrified me. I didn't like that. I thought I was so smart because I hid my eating disorder from my family and my boyfriend on the outside. In here they watch you constantly. Being locked up forced me to be with myself, which terrified me even more. It is getting easier and the other people in here are unbelievably supportive."

"I'm Justin and I'm an anorexic-bulimic and a laxative abuser. This program is really hard. I have been in here for four weeks. The hardest thing for me has been the honesty thing. I have always blamed others for what I have done to myself. I am learning to see what my part has been and I know that I can only change myself. I hope you come in, Kerry."

I did think that I would just stay in my room and go to a few meetings when I felt like it. That heart doctor practically told me I had to live like an invalid anyway. I told myself that I'd tell my AA sponsor about the eating disorder when the time was right. She was overweight after all and I didn't think she'd understand. She did understand about the neighbor who did things to me when he was drunk. I hate him for that. I hadn't told my parents. That is all they would have needed. When I first agreed to come into the program, I thought that secretly I'd still get to have things my way. I thought that if I held out for a little longer, my parents would let me do what I wanted. I think that I hadn't realized how isolated "getting my own way" had made me. I dropped out of college. My friends gave up on me. Even my best friend since the third grade didn't call me anymore. We were blood sisters. I miss her a lot. My recovery has not been able to heal that relationship yet.

I still remember the day that I checked into the unit. The nurses who led me through the admission process asked me so many questions that I didn't want to answer. Of course, I couldn't respond with much emotion: I was completely numbed out from not eating for three days. That night I tried to think back on how I got there. I remember shouting in the mirror, "See what you have done now, stupid!"

But now, so much has changed. I have even helped talk to other girls about the treatment. It sounds so strange to hear myself say it, but I am the one now who says to others, "I really hope you come into the program."

KERRY TRULY HAD COME a long way. When we first met her, she had an incredible strength gained from her battle with alcoholism. She had identified the sexual molestation, which she was no longer keeping a secret from her therapist. She also had a potentially tragic weakness that came from her inability to face her severe eating disorder. Interconnections between eating disorders and chemical dependencies will be intertwined in the stories of these three women. Now, we will introduce you to Amanda.

Amanda, like Kerry, was admitted first through the emergency room. Her husband, Doug, brought her in after she collapsed. She was a middle-aged professional woman and mother of two who had been starving herself and abusing laxatives and over-the-counter diet pills for years. She had had a heart attack six months before we met her. When the doctor questioned her about having an eating disorder, she simply lied, denying she even knew what he was talking about. Recently, things had become worse. Amanda had discovered methamphetamine and had become acutely addicted. She found to her almost fatal and masochistic delight that while high on meth, she could go days without eating. The drug killed her hunger pangs and gave her the energy to get through the day. For a while, her family had no idea what was wrong with her because she did eat in front of them when she had to. Later, in the privacy of her nightly shower, she would simply purge whatever nutrients she had consumed for the sake of her morbid dinner performance.

These diseases tell women that they should feel free to hide their destructive behaviors because "no one will ever find out as long as I don't tell." This is what Amanda thought. But these diseases lie.

These diseases ravage the mind and body, and eventually the whole world can see their ugly truth. Perhaps it's better if we let you see this truth through Amanda's eyes. While Kerry's story is ultimately written from a post-recovery perspective, in Amanda's tale we want to show you the intense denial that diseases can command in their victims. Although Amanda was one of the most acute cases we encountered, she was also among the most tenacious and adamant in refusing treatment until it was almost too late.

### AMANDA

My doctor told me this morning that some nurse named Sandy is coming to talk to me about being in the eating disorder program. My doctor hopes that I will be able to do it now that I'll be willing to do the program "in good faith," as she says. Honestly, I don't know if I will or not. Everyone here thinks I'm sick, but I think hospitals make you sick, so why should I agree to come to one?

I don't really remember arriving on the unit. I must have been in pretty bad shape, or maybe it was the meth I snorted. I have been here about five days. At least, that is what I have been told. I have been eating my meals with them watching me. I manage to hide the butter from some of the staff. I have to. I've always been lactose intolerant, ever since I was a little girl. No one here believes me. They all say I am sick and that I need to get better.

I suppose part of me does think something might be wrong. Six months ago, I had a heart attack and ended up in intensive care. When I came to, I remember lying and telling the doctors that I didn't know why it happened. I promised my husband that I would take better care of myself by eating right but, honestly, I don't know what brought on the attack. I think that some people in my family have had heart trouble. So, maybe it was bad genes. No one ever knew about the laxatives and the diet pills. But they wouldn't understand. I felt so bloated and fat. Here they won't give them to me and I swear that I'm going to burst open like a sausage.

After the heart attack and a stint in ICU, I went home, and two days later I was back on the diet pills. The laxatives started soon after. I had pills stashed in my panty drawer. I was eating some food. I swear that I was making an attempt to get better. Three weeks later, my boss welcomed me back to work. I loved my job. I was sure that working again would help me set my mind straight. But there was always that pressure to be thin. I made so many promises to so many people the day I got out of the hospital, to stay well and to take care of myself. I was so convincing that I believed myself.

At work, my routine soon became my old pattern of "staying up" with the help of diet pills and coffee. The laxatives gradually went up to 60 a day. I didn't eat all day, and I would tell people at work that I had plans to eat at night with my husband. I told my husband that I had a big lunch at work. If I did have to eat with him, I would purge as soon as possible. Once a month my husband would travel and that would be my time to lose control completely. I would binge and purge for hours. My chest would hurt and I would ignore the pain. When I heard my husband coming home from a trip, I would be in bed exhausted, barely able to say good-night. The next morning, I would start all over.

I knew that some people at work would party with drugs and pot on the weekends. I remember looking down on them. In fact, I hated them and wondered when my bosses would fire them for being junkies. But then one Friday night after work, someone offered me methamphetamine while we were at an office happy hour. I was hungry and in such pain with stomach cramps that even the booze wasn't making me feel better. I said yes to the offer. I took the methamphetamine and with my friend instructing me, I snorted it up my nostrils. Nothing hurt anymore. I wasn't hungry and I felt full of energy. I left the bar having bought one bag from my "junkie" coworker with the promise to buy another from her later in the week. From that moment, I was convinced that I had found the "solution" to my problems.

Only a couple months later, people at work had the nerve to tell me that I looked horrible. They started asking me why I looked so bad, why I always had black circles under my eyes. My hair started to fall out by the handfuls. I was having trouble concentrating. I was dozing off at work, in the middle of conversations, at dinner. Nothing helped, not the diet pills, not the meth. My husband questioned me over and over again. Over and over again, I lied. How could all of this be related to eating anyway? I was eating all the time. I ate. You saw me eat. Even if later at night I would bring it all back up. But I couldn't keep it down. It wasn't that I wanted to puke. My body was telling me that it had been overstuffed, that it needed to feel free to breathe. My family has bad genes. The women in my family are fat. I was sure that my problems stemmed from some other cause, some undiagnosed disease that ran in my family that the swarms of stupid doctors I have seen have failed to diagnose. It's probably some sort of food allergy.

The day my husband and my boss did the intervention was surreal. My husband said our marriage was in trouble, and my boss said that I couldn't come back to work until I was healthy. They said that I had hit bottom. When they said it, I just did not have the strength to resist. I guess I was willing to come into treatment and sign the papers. It's pretty foggy. I still am not sure that I belong here. I mean, what kind of a hospital will give a patient butter when she has already told them that she is lactose intolerant? I also wish I could do one more hit of meth. Just to give me the energy for treatment and clear my head.

Here comes the nurse. I know I could just tell her what she wants to hear. I am good at that. Right now, I am not sure what I'm going to do. Something doesn't feel right, but I don't know what it is.

AMANDA GRUDGINGLY AGREED TO stay for the treatment that everyone around her knew she needed. It would be weeks into the recovery process, however, before she would be able to admit freely that she actually needed our help. Although Amanda was not primarily a drug addict, once introduced to the drug, she quickly became a regular and desperate user. Her newfound addiction to the drug was a perfect accomplice for her already out-of-control eating disorder. Blow by blow, the disorders conspired to destroy her mentally and physically. The meth helped her hide the immediate effects of her eating disorder and the eating disorder became a constant source of excuses to fuel her drug intake. Consider how "sneaky" these diseases truly are: Although she was at the end of her rope physically and mentally when she arrived in our care, she continued to suggest that there was a mistake, that food allergy was the cause of her deterioration.

Not all of our patients are in denial as deeply as Amanda. In fact, some patients come to us willingly, even desperately, wanting us to intervene in the chaos of their disorders. One such patient was Heather. Heather was in her late 20's. Unlike Kerry and Amanda, she had not truly reached rock bottom. Nevertheless, Heather could read the writing on the wall and she knew that it was only a matter of time. Heather realized that she was both a bulimic and an alcoholic. Sometimes, treatment professionals will add the term "functional" to the diagnosis of Heather's condition. We think that term is profoundly misleading. After all, no one talks about "functional breast cancer" or "functional liver disease" or "functional osteoporosis" or even a "functional dog bite" that has clipped a major vein. No, bulimia and alcoholism are progressive and ultimately fatal conditions that, if left untreated, will kill their victims. Even though Heather had not reached rock bottom, we would not call her functional. Perhaps the best rebuttal against the use of the term is how we like to describe Heather's current situation: a recovering alcoholic/bulimic who is thriving. You are going to find Heather funny, intelligent and insightful. You need to realize that sharp wit and a good sense of humor do not inoculate you against these diseases though. For all of her smarts and wit, Heather still needed to seek treatment to regain control of her life.

### HEATHER

I'm Heather and I am an alcoholic. I'm Heather and I am a bulimic. I'm Heather and I'd like a Greek omelet with wheat toast and a Bloody Mary, extra spicy. I tried not to smirk too much. That's how this place works, right? I thought that I'd start the recovery ball rolling and get myself in with the nurses. From where I was sitting, they looked like the neighborhood pack of strays and any bone I could throw them might help sweeten them up. Apparently, they failed to get the good-natured irony. Maybe it was brewery breath? Maybe it was the blood-shot eyes? What were they expecting anyway? They were the ones who insisted on an 8:00 A.M. admission on Saturday morning. They refused to bring me an eye-opener and my hands began to shake.

I knew for a long time I was out of control. I had charmed my way into the perfect job. I was a sales director for a major corporation, and one of my main duties was wining and dining clients at power luncheons. I would get toasted three or four times a week with top executives. It's not like they weren't throwing them back, too. It's just that somehow I always had one or two more than they did. Then I realized I could just work this into my sales pitch, especially with the men. I'd just giggle and say, "I'm so embarrassed. That martini went right to my head. That's never happened before." Men love to feel in control so it actually would help me seal the deal.

Last week, I guess I stepped over the line though. Someone reported me to my boss. Probably one of those little witches whose sales aren't as high as mine. Women forget we're to back one another. My boss called me in and said that I was "endangering the company's good reputation." I had to do some fast moves to get out of that one. First, I made sure to cry when he gave me the lecture on the dangers of drinking too much. I apologized so sincerely and lied about a member of my family being terminally ill. All was forgiven. I walked away thinking, "Damn I'm good." I went out that night with some of my drinking buddies from another office. I got completely smashed. I claimed that I was toasting my success but, really, I was trying to dull that tug in the pit of my stomach. Guilt, denial, self-destructive behavior, it was all down there in a tight knot.

The bulimia really started when I was in high school. I was always outgoing, friendly, funny, the center of attention. I guess you'd say that I was one of the popular people. My passion was sports and I played soccer from the age of five. I met Kyle at the beginning of junior year. He sat behind me in American History. At first, he'd just make this stupid joke about us going out. He'd act as if we already were together and start making these crazy plans for prom. Eventually, it sort of worked. I wanted to go out with him. He was funny and paid a lot of attention to me. I hadn't dated much and was attracted to him. My friends hated him and told me he was trouble. Somehow, all that just made me want to go out with him more.

My parents never liked him either. They could never point to anything specific. They just didn't like him. The next thing you know, we were spending all our time together. Looking back, the more time we spent together, the creepier he got. He wanted me to quit soccer because he didn't want to be lonely. In some screwed up way, I thought that was sweet and that it meant that he "loved me." I kept playing anyway, but still Kyle got more and more demanding.

Then he started to be angry all the time. He'd say mean things about the way I looked. The worst was, "You eat like a pig and pretty soon you are going to look like a pig. Oink! Oink! Piggy!" I solved that problem by letting my binge eating and vomiting, as usual, help me through the crisis. For a while at least, I even thought that it was working, that it really was solving the problem. After all, he was never the wiser and he started to compliment me on losing weight. I thought if I were thin then he'd be nicer to me. Somehow, that never happened. He'd compare me to other girls constantly. I always came up short. I now realize that I was becoming quieter and more and more introverted. My self-esteem was flushing down the drain. My whole world revolved around Kyle. I didn't see my friends. All I had was my dirty little secret: bulimia. In some totally messed up way, I thought that the bulimia was the only thing that was truly there for me.

Kyle and his friends started drinking on the weekends in the middle of our junior year. My father was a heavy drinker when I was young so I always said I would not drink. It wasn't unusual for me to drive Kyle and me home after a party. I always worried about him getting himself home. A couple of times, he passed out in my driveway and I had to come up with an excuse for my parents. At times, he became a mean drunk and at one party he was especially cruel to me in front of his friends. To get back at him, I asked another boy for a beer and I never turned back.

We both signed up for the same college 200 miles from our hometown so that family wouldn't be showing up unexpectedly. We practically moved in together as soon as I said goodbye to my folks. The really heavy drinking started on the weekends. He was amused that "miss goody two shoes" was finally loosening up and being more fun around his buddies. The breakup happened when I found him with another girl. He was so drunk and he just laughed at me. I cursed him out and went home with one of his loser friends.

The next day was the first time that I resolved to get my life back together. I stopped returning Kyle's phone calls. I vowed to get serious about school. I slowed down on the drinking. Still, I did return full force to my first love, bulimia. I'd go to the dorm cafeteria and binge on stuff from every food station they had. Then I'd find a place to purge. I'd even raid the refrigerators on every floor of our building and lie like a trooper about not knowing what happened to the food.

I didn't date anyone else. One night, a girlfriend talked me into going to a frat party. Some little witch came up and asked me how Kyle was doing. I immediately went for the booze. I also woke up in someone's dorm room in bed with some drunk whose name I didn't know. That became too familiar a pattern.

After college, I bounced around and then found the company that I'm working for now. Again, I tried to get my act together and for a while it worked. I put my heart into it and got great promotions. I was finally promoted to sales vice president. Even though I was strong for a while, eventually the client lunches and the socializing after work got to me. I didn't want to admit I couldn't drink. I just didn't want to be an alcoholic. Recently, the bulimia has gotten worse than ever.

I have been bulimic for nine years and alcoholic, I guess, from my first drink. I want help.

Unfortunately, Heather's situation is not uncommon. She has known for a long time that she needed help. But she has also been smart enough, clever enough, charming enough and quick enough to improvise coping strategies that have helped her practice both of her diseases. We believe that patients like Heather will never get better as long as they simply try to make it on their own. It makes all the sense in the world that she would have to enlist the support of others. After all, the numbers two-to-one are against her because she's fighting bulimia and alcoholism. Many times, our personalities are double-edged swords. For Heather, her wits and humor for years helped her mask and prolong her destructive behaviors. Through the course of her treatment, she was able to resurrect the positive powers of these traits and use them to honestly explore the painful realities of her life.

## Piecing the Big Picture Together

"Cathy, do you have a minute?"

"How can I help you, Sandy?"

"I have been thinking and want to run some of my thoughts by you. A fair number of our eating disorder patients, sometimes up to 50 percent or more, seem to have significant drug and alcohol problems. Do you think they could benefit from your program too? Would you at least give them an assessment to see what you think?"

"I don't know, but I will be glad to take a look and get back with you."

"Let me tell you some of Kerry's history. She has been clean and sober from drugs and alcohol for almost two years. When Kerry did get into recovery, her eating disorder started to get worse. She refused to eat to the point of some pretty significant heart damage that ended her up on the cardiac unit. She really didn't want to come into the eating disorder program. She came to get her parents off her back. Perhaps not eating became her drug of choice?"

"I'll try and see her later."

My thoughts kept going back to what Sandy had discovered and started thinking about all the addicts and alcoholics who had some type of difficulty with eating, as well. I wanted to choose my words carefully with Kerry because it's bad enough to deal with an eating disorder, let alone another addiction, such as substance abuse.

"Hi, I'm Cathy Napier. Kerry, your doctor wants me to talk with you about your drug and alcohol history."

"There isn't any problem there. I go to an AA meeting every day and I call my sponsor every day. I also am working on the steps. I'm good." I realized that Kerry was having some difficulty dealing with both addictions at the same time.

"Kerry, I am hearing that you are working a strong program for drugs and alcohol. I have two thoughts. You would be a real strength to attend my program in the evenings and share how you are able to stay clean and sober from drugs and alcohol. My second thought is, aren't you curious about how to use your 12 Steps to get into recovery for your eating disorder? Real recovery is to free you from addictions that mask your true feelings. I believe you may be using anorexia as a drug." I paused to allow the reality of my statement regarding total recovery to sink in. "Are you willing to come to my group?"

"I'll come, but can't promise I will stay in it."

"Well, that's a start."

Two weeks later, Sandy approached me again.

"Cathy, I want you to see another patient."

"Sure."

"We have another patient on the eating disorder unit who is also alcohol/drug addicted. She has been drinking and using diet pills. Most recently, she started using methamphetamine. I thought she could benefit from your program. I know Kerry had a real turn-around when she started attending your program, too."

"Sure," I said. "I will be glad to do an assessment and invite her to the evening program."

"Great, I'll get an order from her doctor," replied Sandy

"Let me know and I'll see her today."

"If you have a minute, let me tell you a little bit about her history and what she has been doing so far. Amanda is 42 years old and not very open to treatment. She arrived kicking and screaming on the unit. Her eating disorder consisted of not eating for days and living on coffee and diet pills. She drinks almost daily and has recently used methamphetamine to help her curb her appetite. When she does eat, it's usually in the evening with her husband. Unfortunately, she is an expert at finding ways to purge. Her heart is compromised due to a heart attack six months ago. She lied to her doctor in intensive care about having an eating disorder. This woman is in denial."

The next afternoon, I called Amanda out of her eating disorder group therapy session.

"Amanda. I would like to see you for an assessment, is that okay?" Amanda reluctantly agreed to the assessment.

"Amanda, how much alcohol do you drink?"

"I only drink when I have to entertain clients that I work with."

"Do you use drugs of any kind?" Amanda looked away and started to cry. Her voice started to escalate.

"I'm not a druggie, and I resent you even implying that I am." I could see that she, like most patients, was not ready to address both addictions, so I confronted her.

"Amanda, your intake assessment said that you use diet pills and most recently started using methamphetamine." Again, in denial, she answered defensively.

"I'm here because I have food allergies. My doctors don't understand that I've had them all my life. I need to learn to eat the right food, that's all!"

I needed her to really hear what I was saying, so I very sternly said, "I think you're in gross denial or you want to hold onto the drugs as you would hold on to a security blanket. I'm going to suggest you attend the evening chemical dependency program. Face it Amanda, you're an addict and an alcoholic."

"I don't like you and you're wrong!" she shouted, and then she walked out of my office, slamming the door behind her. I had just witnessed another patient who has been using chemicals to aid and abet the eating disorder. The good news is that she was willing to come to my program.

I turned my chair around away from my desk. As I looked out the window over the downtown skyline, my thoughts were about Kerry and Amanda. My mind raced over the many years I had been seeing patients. I thought about the alcoholic who had always stated that food interfered with the ability to get high so they wouldn't eat. The methamphetamine and cocaine addict who would go for days without eating because they had no appetite. Now, the eating disorder patient has crossed my path using alcohol and drugs to help her sustain her eating disorder. Patients were not getting into recovery because we weren't treating all addictions at the same time. Bingo! I rushed out the door to find Sandy.

"Hey, we've stumbled onto something here."

"I know," she said. "These women hold onto other addictions that soon get them into relapse. We've minimized the drug and alcohol usage in the past. We've wondered why the relapse rate is so high with eating disorder patients."

"Well, now we know why," I said.

After several meetings regarding the patients we had treated over the past few months, we were able to see them benefiting from the treatment of both diseases.

We were continuing to assess patients identified as dually addicted.

The next patient sent to me for an assessment was Heather. Sandy recounted that Heather brought herself to treatment because she was ready to get help. She was really charming but quite sick. She is bulimic and an alcoholic, but no drugs that we were aware of. Sandy's assessment indicated that Heather was not as ready as she thought she was but we gave her credit for bringing herself to treatment. We both agreed that the patients were getting better quicker when we treated both addictions simultaneously. We were excited about the developments that we were witnessing and Sandy suggested that we should write a paper together. "Paper? How about we go for the whole ball of wax and write a book."

"Oh sure, dream big, Napier."

That is how the idea for a book came into being, with Sandy approaching me to do an assessment on one of the eating disorder patients. I didn't know that much about eating disorders but, very quickly, I came to appreciate that an addiction is an addiction. These young women became a favorite population with me because of their potential, and when they got the connections, they really got it. Sometimes, in fact, they got into recovery for their drugs and alcohol before they did for their eating disorders. Yes, some of them refused to admit that alcohol was a problem and they were calling me three months later from college saying that they were getting drunk every day and could I help them. It is just so hard for them to think that they can never drink again at 18 or 19 years old. Finally, I learned to tell them to get a year of recovery from the eating disorder under their belts and then maybe they could revisit the alcohol.

Within 48 hours, as is the protocol, I was meeting with Heather.

"Heather, could I see you for a few minutes? Your doctor wants me to do an assessment on your use of drugs and alcohol. Are you agreeable?" She was somewhat hesitant, but followed me to my office. Heather's assessment was accurate in determining that she was another patient who had a dual addiction. Heather agreed to treat both addictions at the same time. She ended up after treatment attending Alcoholics Anonymous on a regular basis.

## Assignment for Chapter Three

### PSALM 139

God, you have probed me, you know me:
You know when I sit and stand;
You understand my thoughts from afar.
My travels and my rest you mark;
With all my ways you are familiar.
Even before a word is on my tongue,
God you know it all.

## Quote

"Emotion is the chief source of all becoming conscious. There can be no transforming of darkness into light and of apathy into movement without emotion."

Carl Jung

## Meditation

1. Get into a quiet place.
2. Center your thoughts on emotions that you have not felt in some time due to the overpowering addiction in your life.
3. Slowly, say part of the quote that would lead you into getting in touch with your emotions. For example, do you feel any calm or peace about getting into recovery from an eating disorder and/or substance abuse disorder? Do you feel more love toward your family for being supportive in this step toward your recovery? Are you getting to know yourself better as result of being in recovery?
4. Ask for guidance from a Higher Power to help you get in touch with other emotions.

## Commentary

When we ask God to reveal ourselves to us, we need to be prepared for the discovery because He knows us better than we know ourselves, as we learn in Psalm 139. When we get away to a quiet place with Him to commune, we can expect to have our emotions come into play stronger than ever. Thus, the passage that states, "Be still and know that I am God." His power and love reveals to us our innermost thoughts. We just need to relax and allow them to surface. Take the knowledge that has been discovered and apply it to our recovery.

Once you become clean and sober, you start to realize that addiction is total darkness with no light. This condition is depression, which occurs over time when using alcohol and drugs and having an eating disorder surface into nothing but a life full of darkness. We have to feel hope in order to move from addiction to recovery, from darkness into light.

There has to be some comfort in knowing that you have support from your loved ones as you get into your recovery journey. The addict needs to know that families get sick, too, so addiction affects the entire family system. We have put together specific written assignments for a family wellness program in our next chapter. Remember that there should be no secrets when trying to recover from addiction, so family members and patient, please approach the following chapter with an open mind.

FOUR

# Fitting Families Into the Big Picture

**CHAPTER OBJECTIVES**

- ✓ *Families will be equipped with clear direction on how to administer self care techniques.*
- ✓ *They will participate in a family exercise.*
- ✓ *They will learn how to not feel guilty.*

*We believe you.*, the family, should be included in the simultaneous approach and integrated treatment of your loved one who may suffer from an eating disorder and/or substance abuse. We believe your family involvement is vital to the wellness of your family member. The disease has affected the entire family so it makes sense to treat the family unit as well. Families fall on a spectrum of being quite healthy to being quite unhealthy, which oftentimes masquerades as huge family secrets. To be able to speak openly and honestly in a safe setting wherever a particular family falls on the spectrum, without a judging attitude, is a goal of any family work. Teenagers are still dependent on their parents for emotional and financial help. In our country, the mean age a young adult leaves home, completing his or her task for independence, is 25. If the milestones of independence are not achieved in early adulthood, the work will still be there to do in her 30's, 40's or 50's. If, at the age of 50, an individual continues doing family of origin work, and they have a spouse and children of their own, then the treatment team could make that observation and guide them to do current work.

When addiction is part of the big picture, the chances of becoming a functioning young adult change radically. One of the hooks for practicing an eating disorder is to remain childlike and dependent—not to grow up. Chemical dependency further complicates the picture. We are now going to talk directly to your family members. You may be curious and want to eavesdrop on what we are going to say:

Thank you for supporting your family member struggling with the deadly addictions of eating disorders, alcohol and drug abuse. Among those suffering mental illness, eating disorders are the number one cause of death. When chemical dependency is added to the mix, the results are truly frightening. Your family members may have major depression or another psychiatric diagnosis that will also be treated.

As a family member, the first question on your mind may be, "Did I cause the eating disorder and/or chemical dependency?" The good news is, no, you did not cause the addictions. The second part of that answer is that you are part of the story to be explored. It may be significant to look at the genetic makeup of your family. Are there other addictions in the family tree? This exploring is to gain understanding. In both Cathy's and Sandy's family picture, addictions were rampant. Cathy lost 16 family members to addictions and Sandy can trace four generations of disordered eating with a strong link to alcoholism, too.

Addictions have many sources. We believe addiction is biological, psychological and social. Therefore, we believe in treating the whole person. Cathy has identified a definite family genetic history of alcoholism and drug addiction going back to her grandparents' heritage. She has been able to trace the family genetic marker of addiction to her Scotch-Irish grandfather and American Indian grandfather. Sandy has been able to trace her eating disorder back generations as well.

Genetic research has given us wonderful news that addictions are definitely biological and not bad behavior. The gene for alcoholism has been identified and researchers are currently working on the genetic markers for eating disorders. It will be a helpful assignment for family members to identify addiction in the family and extended family. These addictions can be eating disorders, chemical dependency, work, sex, gambling—the list goes on.

The worship of the fertility figures of our early ancestors has been replaced today with worship of the runway models as our highest standard of beauty, one to be accomplished at all costs. Our cultural norm for beauty sends a dangerous message to our most vulnerable young who are over-stimulated by the media with this idealized female form (The fact that pictures in magazines are airbrushed is not information our young are willing or able to assimilate.). Stimulant drug use also gives the promise of attaining the "look." Drinking will make it easier to purge to remain thin. By college, the message is that "everyone drinks." Parents may unwittingly play into the notion that young people are just going through a phase. Most young adults will move through late teens and early 20's successfully. We work with the population that is not just going through a phase but who are into deadly addictions.

Exciting research at the University of Pittsburgh by Dr. Walter Kaye has shown that eating disordered women and men were often anxious as young children. Perfectionism was part of their makeup.

They were harm-avoidant children, not wanting to cause waves in the family. They were not the ones typically who were seeking attention. Another sibling may have acted out and put stress on the family, so the young child just had to be a "good" child. Depression can also be part of the picture at an early age.

The patients we work with are intelligent, gifted women. Many of the patients we work with are top athletes on full college scholarships for soccer, tennis, swimming and track. These women athletes practice exercise bulimia along with their anorexia. Exercise is another way in which they purge. They exercise to the point of exhaustion and if they do it, they will usually purge or stick with power drinks. Academically, they are in the upper echelons. Many are natural-born leaders. It is very difficult to understand how these women get caught up in these destructive addictions that compel them to sacrifice their very lives.

The family system may be such that it wasn't a good fit for the particular young woman. Three other siblings may have sailed through the family and did just fine. But, for whatever reasons, including her personal makeup, this woman did not thrive in the family. Sandy, in her story, talks about not being a good fit in her family of origin.

There may have been trauma in the family or outside the family that affected these women greatly. The family meeting at which trauma is first addressed should be addressed at a deeper level with a family therapist after the trauma is uncovered.

How is the family work done? There are highly effective models in different programs. The goal for family work is to talk openly about the family dynamics and then for individual members to share their feelings with one another. We have heard the work being called resentments, regrets and requests; or resentments and regrets; or truth in love. Whatever the work is called, the goals would be similar.

Your job will be to look at your role in her family story. The effectiveness of the family work that we are going to call resentments and regrets will be lost if anyone plays the "blame game." Instead, we invite you to be a family storyteller. Your perspective on the family is valuable. If we only hear from the patient or only hear from one family member, the family story is incomplete. If the individual is married and has children, the work will include the spouse and children who are old enough. Sibling input and work is some of the best work. They can validate the family happenings. It does not matter so much that everyone recall the exact details alike, but that family members are talking to each other directly and that they have an opportunity to hear the painful feelings of the other. It is also important for the other to hear the amends being made in good faith.

Family members, you will really need to take care of yourselves during this process. We encourage you to go to Al-anon to learn about self-care and addictions. In Al-anon, you will learn about support versus enabling. The eating disorder program's weekly education group provides a forum for you to ask questions and to be supported by other families going through the process of supporting a family member in early recovery. We also encourage family members to go see a therapist if some of your own issues come up and you need additional support. If you have an untreated addiction that is affecting the family, what an opportune time to get the help you deserve.

Part of the philosophy we believe in is to have "listening ears." We learned about treating eating disorders and chemical dependency by listening to the women we were treating. Now it is your turn to learn this skill with your family member. In the resentments and regrets exercise, the overall goal is to have families listen to each other doing a scripted exercise that is about expressing feelings.

The eating disorder and the alcohol and drug abuse will both be addressed. The setting is safe and confidential. Let us begin:

In this exercise, the patient and the family members have an opportunity to express feelings directly to each other within the context of a controlled, supportive script and environment. The patient and the family member sit in chairs facing each other in the center of the group. We want the woman with the eating disorder and chemical dependency issues to find her voice and not act out feelings with self-destructive behaviors. The patient writes out her resentments, which are behaviors the family members have done that she resents. The feelings associated with the resentments are also shared. Then the patient makes amends by sharing behaviors that she has done and regrets. She shares the feelings she has about behaving that way. When the patient finishes her work, she sits and listens to the family member share his or her work. They do not respond to each other while the work is being read. When they have both completed the work, they return to their respective seats within the larger group.

The final part of the exercise will include a group process of the work. It is not helpful to go over the work point by point. We have found it helpful to ask the patient and family member if there were any surprises. Most of the time, there are not any surprises. Each party knew the shared information, but it just wasn't talked about, or it was talked about to death. The feelings associated with the event are the gemstone of the activity. After the patient and the family member discuss the experience, the group members are encouraged to give supportive feedback. Supporting the participants for their courage and honesty helps with the healing.

What a gift to the family group to have a parent who has done 12 Step work or who has been in his or her own long-term therapy. We had a wonderful example of that type of parent work with a husband and wife who had been active in Al-anon for years. The mother said, "We realized the wisdom of changing playmates and playgrounds. We were playmates, and we had to change our behaviors using Al-anon wisdom." They were the best example we had witnessed of loving detachment and self-care.

Many times, families have enmeshment issues. Webster's defines enmeshment as: "to catch or entangle in or as if in meshes." After all, if we have done a good job as parents, our children leave us to become their own person on their own spiritual journey. The relationship then is one between adults who love and support each other. When enmeshment is present, the young adult gets "bogged down" in the family issues to their detriment by not getting on with age-appropriate milestones. Enmeshment may be between mothers and daughters or between fathers and daughters. At times, the parental dyad is not strong and alliances between the child and the parent become non-adaptive for the young woman. We see a red flag when we hear that she had a perfect family growing up. We are also concerned when we hear that her mother is her "best friend." We are concerned when the mother tells the daughter everything, especially about her relationship with her husband.

Other times, families may have been overindulgent with the young woman. Some young women have not ever dealt with the word "no," and they may become experts at splitting and manipulating their parents to get their own way. This behavior will not serve them well in the long run. We believe that limits are healthy and necessary.

At the other end of the spectrum, we see examples of neglect. We see young women who have been little adults for a long time and have assumed the responsibility of raising siblings and managing the home. We have heard of children from a very young age being responsible for opening cans to feed themselves and not having a nurturing adult mother provide meals. Because of their role in the family, they miss out on being teenagers and going through the developmental milestones that are age appropriate.

The spectrum that includes the indulgent family, the neglectful family, as well as all the families in between, may not have been able to meet the emotional needs of the child maturing into a young woman or man. We do believe that parents want good things for their children and that they do the best they can with the information they have at the time. Their desire to parent may have been compromised if the parent has an untreated addiction himself or herself. In the education group, we invite everyone to seek the help they deserve.

A phenomenon we are becoming more aware of, working in this field, is the transferring of eating disorders and chemical dependency from one generation to another without anyone trying to break the cycle. We have recognized the genetic component of alcoholism for many years. Forward strides are being made with the genetic component with eating disorders. Over and over, we hear of mothers who were always on a diet. We hear of young women stealing their mother's diet pills. We hear of mothers who are self-loathing of their bodies. We also hear of grandmothers who set up patterns in their homes that proved to be a breeding ground for eating disorders. This could include patterns of overeating on a daily basis and all the women in the family being obese.

We also hear of the father being critical of his wife's body in front of their young daughters. We tell parents not to make comments about their daughters' bodies. We suggest to family members what to say when their daughter asks, "Do I look fat?" There isn't a right answer. This question would indicate that the young woman has some feelings that have been condensed into a "fat thought." Family members can refer the woman to call a support person in recovery to discuss their body image or suggest that body image would be a great topic for her to work on with her therapist in their next session. Family members and support people should always tell the woman what inner qualities of beauty shine forth.

Many times, eating disorders manifest themselves at times of transition. These times could include puberty, high school graduation, beginning college, getting married, having a baby, break up of a significant relationship or losing parents or loved ones. It is common addiction wisdom that emotional growth is stopped at the age the addiction begins. If an eating disorder and/or chemical dependency problem begins at puberty, then the young woman most likely will not be successful at college. Sometimes, these women hold on academically by studying all of the time and isolating from the socialization process. They live in an absorbed world of studying relentlessly and practicing their eating disorder and chemical abuse. They may be binging and purging several times a day, or, if they are starving, they may be living on caffeine and diet pills. Another scenario may be that they get into the party scene and ignore the academic realities. One or more times, they have had to drop out of classes and not finish the semester. Many of the young women come into the program from the physical complications of their bodies giving out from self-starvation, binging and purging, compulsive exercising, and alcohol abuse and drug use.

Because of family issues, it may be recommended that limited family contact be put on the table and discussed. This discussion would occur when the woman is in recovery and her physical condition has been stabilized. This does not mean that these women do not love their families. This does mean that these women are on a sacred journey to embrace their womanhood by freeing themselves from their eating disorder and from chemical dependency. One of our favorite sayings attributed to Ernie Larson is, "If nothing changes, nothing changes." Ernie Larson is well known in the field of addiction recovery. If the family is their only support, then these women do not have the wonderful opportunity to expand their world to include other women in recovery.

Completing resentments and regrets in a group setting can be very powerful. It works best when families attend each week. The different families bond with each other and offer their collective wisdom of experience, strength and hope. The group maintains confidentiality. We have heard from the women that when they start the exercise, the other people in the room fade. The depth of the work does have an effect on everyone and, at times, there are few dry eyes in the room. When the young woman and her family member have finished, they process by sharing back and forth with each other with the guidance of the therapists. The group members also share their observations. The group process becomes greater than the individual experience.

When a parent refuses to come to group or to private therapy to do the work, the woman may choose to do her work with an empty chair. It is not the ideal method, but it can be effective. Many times, a father in the group will speak up and tell the young woman that she did not deserve the treatment she received from her own father. Validation of her experience and her feelings comes from this man speaking up, and it comes from the group. Peers and staff also validate the woman's thoughts and feelings.

In the beginning of treatment, many women say that they have a perfect family. At the time, they do believe that to be so and, from the outside, the family may look healthy. After the woman has been nourished with food and after she has worked through "Can I trust this treatment team?" or "Can I trust this therapist?" we start to hear more honestly about the family. In the next few pages, you will find exercises that are examples of that honesty and act as a guide for the therapist doing family therapy.

# Assignment for the Family Members

## PSALM 91

He that dwelleth in the secret place of the most High shall abide under the shadow of the Almighty. I will say of the Lord, He is my refuge and my fortress my God; in Him will I trust. Surely he shall deliver thee from the snare of the fowler, from the noisome pestilence. He shall cover thee with his feathers, and under his wings Shalt thou trust: his truth shall be thy shield and buckler. Thou shalt not be afraid for the terror by night; nor for the destruction that wasteth at noonday. A thousand shall fall at Thy side, and ten thousand at Thy right hand; but it shall not come nigh thee. Only with thine eyes shalt thou behold and see the reward of the wicked. Because thou hast made the Lord, which is my refuge, even the most High, thy Habitation; there shall no evil befall thee, neither shall any plague come nigh thy dwelling. For He shall give His angels charge over thee, to keep thee in all thy ways. They shall bear thee up in their hands, lest thou dash thy foot against a stone. Thou shalt tread upon the lion and the adder: the young lion and the dragon shalt thou trample under feet. Because He hath set his love upon me, therefore will I deliver him: I will set him on high, because he hath know my name. He shall call upon me, and I will answer him: I will be with him in trouble: I will deliver him, and honor him. With long life will I satisfy him, and show him my salvation.

*Quote*

## A BROKEN FAMILY TREE

I am one of many
Small braches of a broken tree
Always looking to the ones above
For guidance, strength and security.
One branch trying
To keep the others from breaking away
Who will fall?
And who will stay?
Now I stand alone
Looking at the earth through the rain
And I see the broken braches I knew
Scattered about me in pain.
There are those who have taken an axe
To the root of our very foundation
And who have passed this destruction
Down to every new generation.
If I could take that axe
I would toss it deep into the sea
Never to return again
To harm the generations that follow me.
I am one of many
But alone I will go
And plant the new seeds
Where a beautiful tree will grow

By Lori A. Cain

## Commentary

THE ABOVE QUOTES ARE great for imagining each line for your soul food in time of trouble. I don't know anything more heartbreaking than watching a daughter going through the throes of an eating disorder or alcohol/drug addiction. The families and loved ones get so desperate in trying to fix it that they actually become the big enabler. They become so co-dependent that they lose who they are and then the addiction makes them sick too. Unfortunately, you the parent have to love from afar, but always try to be supportive when the son or daughter needs a listening ear. Always try to take care of yourself through these difficult times by seeking support for yourselves. While you're meditating on the above quote and/ or the psalm, imagine your child having a protective covering that is provided by the God that you believe in. Take each line and take it within you, so you'll be able to pull up a line from the quote or verse. This is the soul food that will sustain you through the darkness.

## *Questions*

1. How are you taking care of yourself during this troubling time?
2. List the things you're doing that would be considered enabling.
3. What feelings are telling you that you're being co-dependent?
4. List the changes in you since you found out about the disease?
5. List ways your own personal relationship with your partner has changed.
6. Are you moving closer to your God or higher power or becoming more distant?
7. Please realize this is not your fault, but you are being tortured by guilt. List the things that make you feel guilty.
8. Now you're ready to do the family work with your loved one!

# A Program Exercise for the Family Therapist

## EXPOSING THE FAMILY SECRETS

Below you will find examples of resentments and regrets that you may use as a guide to help you come up with your own personal resentments and regrets. You will need to reach down deep inside yourself, with the help of a family therapist, to explore the resentments and regrets you have harbored for your family members and to take ownership of your part in the family dysfunction. Resents and regrets should only be done with a trained therapist. We suggest that if you're not doing resents and regrets in a treatment facility that you request a therapist do the family work with you.

## DAUGHTER'S RESENTMENTS TO FATHER

> I resent that your work came first and you traveled so much. Our relationship and the family came in second. I felt ignored.
>
> I resent that you spent time with my brother at his sporting events and that you rarely came to mine. I felt jealous.
>
> I resent that you commented on my mother's body and called her fat in front of us kids. I felt ashamed.
>
> I resent that you commented on my body when my body started to mature. I felt ashamed and embarrassed.
>
> I resent that you made rude comments about other women that you saw in public. I felt humiliated.
>
> I resent that you divorced my mother and that you broke up our family. I felt angry.

I resent that you were unaware of my being on drugs and coming home drunk. I felt invisible.

I resent that you spoke poorly of my mother after the divorce. I felt betrayed.

I resent that you put me in the middle of your relationship with my mother. I felt helpless.

I resent your excessive use of alcohol. I couldn't bring friends home because I never knew what kind of mood you would be in. I felt unloved and scared.

I resent that you made me your confidante. I felt used and violated.

I resent that you didn't provide a spiritual base for our home. I felt confused and alone.

## DAUGHTER'S REGRETS TO FATHER

I regret all the lies that I have told you to protect my eating disorder. I feel ashamed.

I regret my irritability and mood swings when you would try to ask me questions. I feel immature.

I regret calling you names and saying that I hated you. I feel ashamed.

I regret driving under the influence of drugs and alcohol. I feel irresponsible.

I regret using your love to manipulate you to practice my addictions. I feel manipulative.

I regret using your money to buy drugs and alcohol. I feel deceitful.

I regret using your money to buy binge foods. I feel ashamed.

I regret that I had to withdraw from college twice. I feel immature.

I regret that I have lost your trust because of my addictions. I feel ashamed.

## FATHER'S RESENTMENTS TO DAUGHTER

I resent the eating disorder and the physical damage that has been done to your body, including the heart damage and bone loss. I feel angry and scared.

I resent the drinking and drug use. I feel angry.

I resent the lies that you used to protect your addictions. I feel betrayed.

I resent the money you have wasted by dropping out of school. I feel used.

I resent you isolating yourself in your room and not being part of the family. I feel sad and cheated.

I resent the mood swings and your irritability when I ask you a question. I feel irritated.

I resent the family events that were dictated by your eating disorder, such as only eating at certain restaurants. I feel used.

I resent that you would not help with family chores. I feel angry.

I resent the disrespect that you showed your mother. I feel angry.

I resent that you do not share with me who you are. I feel cheated.

I resent that you have not lived up to your potential and that you are unable to see the caring, intelligent, funny and wonderfully unique human being that I know you to be. I feel angry.

## FATHER'S REGRETS TO DAUGHTER

I regret that I didn't spend much time with you when you were young. I gave priority to my work. I feel sad.

I regret that just the two of us didn't go out to lunch together or spend special time together. I feel sad for the missed opportunity.

I regret that I didn't attend your sport events, but I did attend your brother's. I feel unfair.

I regret that I didn't tell you more that I love you and that I value the unique person that you are. I feel sad.

I regret that I didn't provide more of a spiritual foundation for you. I feel remorseful.

I regret that I didn't share my personal faith with you. I feel sorrowful.

I regret that I forced my religious views on you. I feel sad.

I regret that I made comments about your body as you were growing up. I feel ashamed.

I regret that I made negative comments about your mother's body in front of you. I feel ashamed.

I regret that I didn't share stories about my childhood with you. I feel lacking.

I regret I didn't share my emotions openly in front of you and give you permission to have your feelings. I feel inadequate.

I regret that you were witness to constant fighting between your mother and me. I regret that we didn't seek counseling sooner for our marriage. I feel remorseful.

I regret that my drinking has gotten out of hand and that you have had to witness my being drunk. I feel remorseful.

### DAUGHTER'S RESENTMENTS TO MOTHER

I resent that you were always on a diet when I was growing up and you told me that I would not get a man if I were fat. I felt confused.

I resent that we had only low-fat food in our home and yet you were overweight. I felt angry.

I resent that you were always focused on your body and that you were self-critical of your body. You called yourself a "fat pig." I felt unsure and sad.

I resent that you made me your confidante and that you would tell me things about my father that I should not have known. I felt violated.

I resent that you expected me to watch my siblings, feed them and get them ready for school. I felt used.

I resent that you used diet pills and that you offered them to me at an early age. I liked the feeling of being high and continued to use them. I felt abused.

I resent that you did not recognize the symptoms of my eating disorder. I felt ignored.

I resent that you did not recognize that I was coming home drunk and high. I felt neglected.

I resent that you did not get help for your depression sooner and that you spent so much time in bed. I felt helpless.

I resent that you did not model how to express feelings in a healthy manner. I felt sad.

## DAUGHTER'S REGRETS TO MOTHER

I regret telling all the lies to practice my eating disorder. For example, telling you that I had eaten when I had not. I feel remorseful.

I regret bingeing and purging in your home. I feel ashamed

I regret being a poor role model to my younger sister or brother and not being involved in his or her life. I feel regretful.

I regret being self-absorbed and not seeing the pain that I was causing you and the family. I feel selfish.

I regret calling you names and being disrespectful. I feel ashamed.

I regret coming home drunk and high and driving under the influence. I feel irresponsible and untrustworthy.

I regret taking your things without asking you because I knew that you would say "No." I feel ashamed.

I regret not coming to you sooner with my problems. I feel manipulative.

I regret having to drop out of school and wasting so much money. I feel irresponsible.

## MOTHER'S RESENTMENTS TO DAUGHTER

I resent all the lies that you told so that you could practice your eating disorder. I feel used.

I resent the physical damage you have done to your body, including the heart damage and bone loss. I feel sad and scared.

I resent the rules that you dictated about which restaurants we could eat at as a family so that you could eat safe foods. I feel violated.

I resent the family celebrations you have ruined because of your eating disorder. I feel angry.

I resent that you were not a positive role model for your siblings. I feel helpless and sad.

I resent your isolating yourself in your room. I feel frustrated and cheated.

I resent the mood swings and irritability in the house. I feel angry.

I resent your bingeing and purging in our house. I feel violated.

I resent the name-calling you used and the disrespect you have shown me. I feel disrespected.

I resent the way you have treated your stepfather. I feel torn.

I resent the alcohol and drug use in our house. I resent that you gave pot to your younger brother. I feel angry.

## MOTHER'S REGRETS TO DAUGHTER

I regret that I was a poor example to you with my own eating habits. I feel irresponsible.

I regret that I was so focused on my physical appearance. I feel superficial.

I regret that I made so many negative remarks about my body. I feel remorseful.

I regret that I was so focused on your appearance and set the stage for you to be focused on your outward appearance. I feel sad.

I regret that I offered you some of my diet pills and that I started you on a diet at an early age. I feel sad.

I regret that I did not see the signs of your eating disorder and alcohol and drug abuse and insist that you seek treatment sooner. I feel foolish.

I regret that I made you my confidant and told you things about your father that you should not have known. I feel foolish.

I regret that I did not get help for my depression sooner and you ended up raising your siblings. I feel neglectful.

I regret that I did not protect you from your stepfather/ father. I feel sad.

I regret not being closer in our relationship. I feel sad.

I regret that I didn't show you more physical affection and tell you everyday that I love you dearly. I feel lacking.

# Assignment for Chapter Four

For the Patient

## PSALM 32:3

As long as I kept silent,
My bones wasted away:
I groaned all the day.

## Quote

When will women begin to have the first glimmer that above all other loyalties is the loyalty to Truth, i.e., to yourself, that husband, children, friends and country are as to nothing to that?"

Alice James (1848-1892), Diary (November 19, 1889)

## Commentary

THIS WORK ON YOUR family is to be done in good faith on both sides. The goal is to have your forum to speak your truth and then to leave the events and feelings in the recovery room and to see the sunshine of each day as a new beginning. To not move on is to ask your addictions to stand by because they will soon be needed to take care of your hurt feelings of "look what others have done to me." This is a clear choice one makes and, of course, your Higher Power is always available to give you the strength for your new way of looking at life. Allow the process to begin and, in your meditation, be open to what your fears may be. Work with your fears not only in your meditation, but with your therapist and treatment team. Be aware of how seductive the voice of your addictions can and will be to keep you stuck in the "same old, same old." Treat yourself with dignity and respect always.

FIVE

# Cathy's Story: How I Gave and How It Changed My Life.

As the cold, damp wet awakens me I'm puzzled to what has happened. My clothes drenched with sweat and the stench of puke is a constant reminder how sick this problem has made me. The smell of vomit hits my nostrils like I had just walked across a landfill. The memory of the evening before is a fog and as much as I try to remember, I can't.

It's the early morning hour and I'm again awakened by the familiar taunting of the demon that's wearing on me. Slowly I pull myself out of bed to the kitchen cabinet where I keep the bottle of gin. I take a swig from the bottle and the insanity of the burning sensation is enjoyable as it slowly goes down my throat. The excitement comes as I tiptoe back to my room, realizing that pretty soon I would get that much-needed sleep.

The morning brought the same life-numbing routine: get up and drink, go to work and drink, go to lunch and drink, come home and drink until bedtime. In my rational moments, I remember how it all started, but always the alcohol and pills kept the recovery only as a mantra in my mind that I would say over and over, "I need to quit…."

I'm driving through Mossy Bottom in the early spring on the way to visit my cousin Barb who is as close as a sister. I have a warm sense of well-being come over me like after meditating. The area was well-traveled by my family when I was a kid growing up in a section of Ashland, Kentucky called Westwood. I arrive late in the evening just as the fog creeps in, leaving a mysterious aura in its hazy path. As I'm driving, my mind drifts back to the days as a young child when life seemed so unimportant and certainly didn't have its chance to taint me. Fond memories were easily recalled, times of pure innocence, the 1950's when the war was long over, enough to at least bask in the peaceful time that everyone in America was enjoying.

I finally arrive at Barb's house just in time to talk for awhile then drop into bed. The next morning, I wake early to the familiar sounds of the country with hundreds of birds welcoming the day or the sound of a rooster crowing. Being back in Ashland after many years of living in Texas and New Mexico was both bitter and sweet for me. As I walk through the familiar woods on this crisp spring morning and as the air flows through my nostrils, it gives me a pleasant sensation of many familiar smells. I'm seeing the trees in these same woods I played in as a child all dressed in their full covering of leaves ready for the summer ahead. The mountain Laurel is a constant reminder that anyone walking through these woods has just reached nature's grand finale. Memories of past years are fresh in my mind, as if they had just happened. I look at where I am today and the long, hard road to get to this place of contentment, that is, contentment with a tinge of pain that has been woven into my mind from the difficulties from the past. My mind goes back decades ago as I remember and tell this story of triumph.

THIS WAS MY TOWN Ashland, Kentucky, a place nestled within a valley surrounded by the foothills of the Appalachian Mountains. A place where I was born, a safe place to grow up and a place I still call home.

I understand the night I was born my father was pulling a three day drunk and didn't show up at the hospital. I was later told he quit after being given an ultimatum by my mother. He attended Alcoholics Anonymous six months after I was born. I never knew him as a drunk, but as a sober dad. He would often talk about his problem with drinking and his recovery with warnings to me about the family problem. I never saw him drink, ever. My dad was a kind man who rarely got upset. He had a fair complexion due to being half Irish and half Scottish. My grandfather was from Scotland and my grandmother was from Mayo County, Ireland. They settled in Virginia and later in Kentucky.

We lived out in Boyd County, which was considered living in the country. The winter months were hard in the country. There was always food due to my mother canning the summer's vegetables and plenty of firewood for the fireplace. The neighbors would give their thoughts about the winter that was surely going to be the worst ever and that was mostly taken out of the Farmers Almanac. They talked about dreading the snow and hard, cold winters ahead. My dread was the pneumonia that I would get every winter. The cough was treated with a down home remedy combination of whiskey, honey and lemon. I was given this on a regular basis with no complaints from me. Even then I liked the taste and the effects. I think I may have even faked a cough or two. My mother didn't realize that she was feeding an addiction with this combination. My earliest recollection of this medication starts at four years old.

I think everyone should live in the country for at least a few years during the early part of their life. I had the opportunity to experience Biology first hand. Our little house sat on a few farm acres that is the area of Westwood called Pine Acres. When I was growing up there was nothing surrounding our house except a few wonderful neighbors and plenty of woods. Faye, my childhood friend, and I played out in the country woods most days until dark. We watched and studied all the creatures that roamed the woods of that little county.

In the country people live differently than in the city. They have to use every bit of nature's gift to live. The term that is often used, living off the land, is so true, because that's exactly how it is. I believe that there's a character-building as a result of eking out a living off the land. There are and there were strange things that happened that I know must have had some negative effect on me. "Come hold this chicken's head," my mother said. I told her no. As quickly as she could, she raised this scary looking butcher knife and chopped off the chicken's head. I couldn't believe what I saw next. Could this be one of the chickens that I gathered eggs from every morning or fed corn to in the late afternoon? There was this chicken hopping around the yard with blood squirting out of its neck while it hopped around. Then finally with what seemed to be forever the poor chicken croaked right there in front of me with blood everywhere. I couldn't have been but four or five years old at the time. I swear this is why today I pass out at the sight of blood.

My mother was a strong woman who could survive off the land. I think somehow, in the back of her mind, she was trying to have me grow up the same way. Perhaps in some way there was some transference of her inner strength passed on to me. She was a beautiful woman. Her skin was as smooth as a baby's behind with a creamy light brown color to it. She had a big head of wavy, jet black hair that would fall down to the sides of her face where her navy blue button eyes looked black next to her hairline. She was full-blooded Cherokee Indian. I would ask, "Are you colored? My friends think that you're a colored woman." Her reply would always be she was "Black Dutch". She never used the term Indian and during that era that was probably a smart thing to do on her part. I was grown before I realized who the black Dutch are in the Native American population. They're Cherokee Indians from the Chickamauga Tribe. They settled in Tennessee, Kentucky and North Carolina.

My grandparents settled in the Cumberland Mountains in a place called Rockhold, Kentucky and are listed on the Dawes roles. The Dawes roles allowed each Native American to be awarded 200 acres of land, and my grandparents, on theirs, built a beautiful farm house, with a huge front porch and a tin roof, so when it rained you could hear the rain tap on the roof. The house was wooden outside and inside with wooden floors throughout the house. In the middle of the living room was a large fireplace that mainly burned coal that my grandpa dug out from his land. Many times when we would arrive for a visit in early spring on a Friday evening and park the car on the road before making the mile trek down the hollow to their house. The spring rains would wash the road out so we would walk the hollow because we were afraid the car would get stuck. The walk was always a pleasant one especially if we were led by the moonlight flowing through the trees. When we arrived I would lie in the living room in a huge featherbed and fight sleep so I too could catch-up on the news. I would hear them talk about the ones who were sick in the family with alcoholism. The term "alcoholism" was never used. They merely said, "Perry, Elvie, George, Lewis, Faye etc. were not doing so well."

When my grandfather died, they sold the farm and my grandmother stayed with each child for a month of two. I remember when it was our turn for her to stay with us. I had to sleep on a pallet on the floor next to her bed because she would sleepwalk, so they wanted her to step on me rather than fall down our stairs. I would lay awake listening to her pray for each of her children. She prayed a lot for Perry, he was the alcoholic who eventually died due to his alcoholism. I couldn't understand anything she was saying, only the names of each child was clear. I thought my grandmother spoke in Pentecostal tongues but instead she was praying in her native tongue. Later I realized why she was a woman of few words because she didn't know a lot of English words. My grandfather was also a man of few words, but I never heard him speak in his native tongue.

We moved into town to get away from the cold, damp winters in the country. My brothers, who were much older than me, would show up for long periods of time throughout my growing up years. They were always cussing, smoking and drinking. They were in and out of the house due to coming home from the service or divorce. Everyone in the house but my mother smoked. Everyone in the house but my father drank. So I naturally thought the vices were not only okay, but really cool. The early lessons learned were smoke, drink, cuss and be as wild as you want because there were no seemingly consequences at the time. Hugh was the oldest and was the hot-tempered one. He came home after his divorce and stayed several years until he married again. One afternoon he came through the back door, slamming the screen door almost plum off the hinges. "Where's the gun? I'm going to blow that sonofbitchin' dog to hell and back." Somehow, our neighbors, the Irving's, huge German shepherd got loose and trapped Hugh between our house and garage. The dog could be intimidating enough from a distance more or less being waist to face with him. Everyone starting screaming, "We have to live here, you can't kill our neighbor's dog." He didn't kill the dog because he couldn't find the gun, not because he had an attack of conscience.

It was tough for my family to adjust to city living. In the country that dog would've already been dead. George was also back due to a divorce from Margie. George had been a POW in the Korean War and suffered from terrible post-traumatic stress. He at one time was extremely good looking, but life had taken its toll on him and he looked much older than his late 30s. George drank and yes was an alcoholic by the time he was 30. As George got older and continued to self-medicate with alcohol, he got crazier. I really didn't put any label on him, because at the time I didn't know anything about mental illness. I just knew that George was strange, as a matter of fact, my entire family was strange. George would sit out in front of our house, which was now in town, not in the country, where sitting with a shotgun over his knee wouldn't have been witnessed by anyone instead of by everyone. I could see cars drive up and down our little residential street with people taking a long look at this guy dressed in a heavy overcoat, long winter pants and hat in the hot humid summer with a shotgun over his lap. I would come home from school with some of my friends and we would step over him as if what was going on was normal. There wasn't anything normal about it. I just didn't know any different and had become immersed in the craziness.

The move into town proved to be beneficial for not only my pneumonia, but for my social network as well. I had my good friend Faye, but she was my only friend in the country. In town, there were kids everywhere. Crabbe Elementary was my grade school up to sixth grade. Diana Judd was one of my best friends in my sixth grade class. The following year we headed for Coles Junior High. There was this cool kid named Mary Tanner who moved to Ashland and attended Coles some time after the beginning of the year. Seems as if Diana already knew Tanner from when they were small children. Tanner left Ashland when she was a small child due to her mother's death from multiple sclerosis and her father's alcoholism. Tanner ended up in an orphanage in a place called LaGrange, Kentucky where the orphanage was located and stayed there until her father sobered up and then she was allowed by the state to move in with him. The child welfare system probably wouldn't have let Tanner go live with her father unless her father was sober and unless the grandmother was in close proximity. The first time I saw

Tanner I thought she was one of the coolest girls I had ever met. She had on a white blouse, a sweater with a ribbon stripe down on one side. The sweater was burnt orange with a horse on it. She also had on an A-line skirt and Bass Weejuns without socks. I think everyone in Ashland liked Tanner's tasteful dress attire. She was considered cool. We were seeing all the girls dress like Tanner. Everyone had an A-line skirt made, because the shops didn't sell them, they didn't know Tanner was coming to town. We could get Weejuns and pretty soon the stores started selling Tanner's famous ribbon sweaters. Even though my name was Catherine, I went by the name of Cathy. Tanner never called me Cathy, she would either call me Napier or "Cathern," but never Cathy.

Coles Junior High became a great place for all of us to develop some wonderful social skills. The school was small enough that we basically knew everyone in all three grades. In our seventh, eighth and ninth grades, we partied everywhere, but mainly in my basement at 813 22nd Street. The basement was converted into a type of kids' den. We had couches and chairs and of course a great record player that played 45's. We played all of Elvis's songs, Roy Orbison, The Big Bopper, Ricky Nelson, and the music of Jackie Robinson. The fast dance was the Jitter Bug and later we just moved to music without holding hands, thanks to Cubby Checker and Jerry Lee Lewis. We had parties in that old basement for at lease three years during our seventh, eighth and ninth grades. We were all too young to drive, so we had to do something on the weekends in order to see one another. During the summer, we hung out more frequently and played all those kissing games that schoolchildren find so risque. One summer, Faye even came to stay with us for several weeks.

One particular day, the summer heat was sweltering like most humid southern towns and on this particular day you could cut the air with a knife. I had just turned 16 and I felt about as grown up as the family that surrounded me. It was a summer yard party at my

Aunt Nora's house on Central Avenue. The house was in the style of the Old South, with red brick walls and miniature white columns and a huge lush green yard in the back. My father and mother was close to my aunt, my dad's sister, and we spent a great deal of time with her in the comfort of that old house. The backyard was always filled with family and friends. Unfortunately, living up to the Scotch-Irish cliché, plenty of liquor of every kind flowed freely. Ironically, my father, a recovering alcoholic, regularly volunteered as the bartender. I don't know how he managed never to take a drink, but to my knowledge, he never did. Family tradition allowed anyone 16 or older to drink and this particular party was my big day. I sauntered over to a washtub full of beer and picked one up as if I had been doing it for years. Little did I realize that I wasn't growing up, but instead had taken my first step down a road of destruction and that it would take decades to find my way again.

I was a junior in high school. The beginning of life, career and happiness, that is, if you don't have an addiction waiting in the wings to rob you of youth and years of preparation for a better life. It seemed like a good year in America too, except for the Vietnam War. A lot of our boys from Ashland who had graduated were being drafted and then deployed to Nam. John F. Kennedy was president. My friends and I tried to imitate his Boston accent and did a poor job of it with our Kentucky twangs, but we tried anyway. It was November right before Thanksgiving when Mr. Ellis came over the loud speaker almost at the end of the day. My fellow Biology students and I were putting our instruments away when Mr. Ellis announced that President Kennedy had been shot and that the President was dead. We all just stood there, too shocked to cry. Then reality sunk in and we started and the tears were heard all through the classroom. I continued to drink and I guess I could've blamed Kennedy's death for that and probably did blame him. I was totally oblivious to the fact that alcohol was controlling me, and that not so good feeling I was having most days was a hangover. I was definitely in denial that I not only looked forward to the next time I would get to drink, but that I actually needed it from time to time. I was never really told that my genetic make-up was loaded with a monster that would come to gobble me up for years and the goal of this intruder was to rob me of everything, and then try to kill me. Even if the information had been so readily available would I have listened?

Drinking wasn't cool, but I drank off and on throughout my senior year, though it was on the sly. I had many close friends and loved socializing with them. Diana Ellen Judd and I had been friends since grade school. Diana and I spent that summer walking through our town park, which was called Central Park. Yes, it looks as if we copied that name from New York's famous park. Diana didn't drink and we were as opposite as oil and water, but we liked each other. Diana was perfect in every way, with a beautiful creamy complexion. We used to say she looked like a china doll. She told me that I had offered her a cigarette, but she declined. I vaguely remember trying to get her to smoke, but, knowing me, I probably did offer her one. We rode the bus one Saturday to Huntington, West Virginia to get ourselves a bathing suit before our summer break. I look back at our little shopping spree and realize that even then Diana was a perfectionist. She wanted to make sure that she would pick the perfect suit. We literally shopped in every department store before she picked a bathing suit that was right for her.

I remember the first day of school my senior year looking for Diana to see if we had any classes together. About halfway through the day the news was out that Diana was pregnant, but no one seemed to know where she was. I remember missing her and grieving the loss of my friend. I thought, this isn't the kind of thing that happens to girls like Diana. I could've named a hundred others that this could've happened to with no surprise to anyone, but not Judd. I asked everyone where I could find her. It was as if she dropped off the face of the earth. I missed her and I knew that our friendship would be different.

Some time later, after Diana disappeared, Tanner called, "Do you want to go shopping with me?" It was spring of our senior year and prom night. Tanner and I needed to pick up a single carnation for our dates. Tanner had a steady boyfriend named Dave Turpin. I was going with Nick Jordan, not my steady boyfriend, but someone to go prom with. We had picked up our dates' carnation at Field's Florist. Mine was red and would fit in the buttonhole of Nick Jordan's white jacket.

Nick Jordan, Bill Tom Alexander and his date, Mary Childers, picked me up at the house fairly early. That was okay because I had been ready for hours. Yes, I was pretty excited about our senior prom. We were going to a few pre-prom parties. When those three picked me up, it looked like they were well on their way to partying before getting me. The car radio was blaring, playing our 60's music. I got in the car and we drove to our first pre-prom party, but parked down the street a ways from the house. Nick, Bill Tom, Mary and I drank gin and Seven-Up before each pre-prom party. When the four of us arrived at the prom, we had to go through the receiving line comprised of the principal, the dean of students, and teachers. We were all four in rare form due to being drunk on our butts. Nick and I headed for the dance floor as did Mary and Bill Tom. Nick and I looked over to see Mary and Bill Tom hanging on one another, just barely able to stand up. I felt a tap on my shoulder. It was our principal, Mr. Ellis, who told us that we, along with Bill Tom and Mary, had to leave the prom because we were drunk. I told him that Nick and I were not drunk, but that they were. I was getting ready to say something like, I've done this many times and I'll guarantee you I'm not drunk. It takes a lot for me to get drunk. Nick and I took Bill Tom and Mary to McClure's restaurant to get them sobered up before the post-prom parties. We ordered enough coffee to speed up any narcoleptic, but they stayed pretty smashed the entire evening. I thought that on Monday morning we would all be expelled from school, but we weren't. As a matter of fact, it wasn't even brought up nor did they call our parents. Of course, all our friends knew we had all spent ten minutes at the senior prom.

In the fall of the next year, I left for college. Drinking in college was acceptable, it just wasn't legal. But like most teenagers, I found a way to get alcohol anyway. My college friends and I drank every weekend and, after a while, that's all that we looked forward to. I wasn't a bad student, but before you knew it, I was skipping class and asking for extensions on assignments. Then I dropped a course and, within the year, I'd left college early. I ended up back in my hometown to try to clear my head, but nothing really changed except my geographical location. I continued to drink and party. Looking back, it seems so clear that drinking, partying and studying didn't mix. Unfortunately, like all alcoholics, I couldn't even see that I was slowly but surely pouring my life down the drain.

Alcoholics have rotten judgment and I should know. So, it might not be surprising to learn that a short time after returning home, I accepted the marriage proposal of a man I barely knew. This was my love story: David was tall, handsome and a lush. David and I eventually married. We left straight from the chapel in Kentucky to drive to Virginia to our new residence. Our families had shoe-polished "Just Married" all over the car and even tied tin cans to the bumper. Two country folk from West Virginia pulled up alongside us at a stop sign and handed us a bottle of Early Times bourbon as a wedding present. We thought we were in heaven. We drank straight out of the bottle and drove all the way to Lynchburg, drunk. Our married life was just two drunks playing house. We worked and we drank, we slept and we drank, we ate and we drank, we cleaned and we drank. Basically, we just drank, so it's no surprise that the marriage was strained. I needed some time away so I decided to visit my family in Ashland for awhile. That first summer, I went back to Ashland to stay with my parents. One evening that I spent "catching up" with Tanner and some of her friends, I knew that we were going to drink the night away. When I arrived at Tanner's friend's house, Janice Joplin's *Me and Bobby McGee* was playing on the record player. Tanner said, "Gawd Napier, I love this song." Tanner continued to sing along with Janice and at times out-singing Janice. We drank the night away. I remember thinking that I should take it easy because in the morning I had plans to go horseback riding with my father. Whatever my little voice of reason said, I merely drank it away. I threw back Jack-and-Cokes until I was hammered. I straggled in late and slept just a few hours before heading out. I had a hangover and dazed, but I was determined to ride anyway. A friend of my father's, who owned a horse farm out in Boyd County, invited us to come see his new horses. We arrived early in the morning and, at the last minute, my father decided not to ride. Instead, he stayed to chat with his friend while I went to the barn to saddle up old Rainmaker. Our friend wanted me to have a try at a new horse and he hollered out, "Why don't you take out Kentucky Pride instead? He's a beauty. You'll find him in the last stall." There wasn't much that I liked more than fast young horses, so I saddled up Kentucky Pride. My friends and family often referred to me as the wild one. I guess if you're pegged the wild one by people who know you, then you've somehow got to live up to that label, which I did many times throughout life with my little helper of booze.

Now, Kentucky Pride was a new horse, so we needed to get used to each other before heading out. This horse seemed as nervous about me riding him as I was about trying to learn him. Underneath my legs, I could feel his jerking sensations, but blew it off as he hadn't been ridden much. I thought that a few laps around the timing track would do the trick. When we trotted, it all seemed good and then, suddenly, the saddle slipped to the left. In my haze from the evening before, I hadn't tightened the saddle strap. The saddle was turning sideways. Kentucky spooked and took off at a gallop. I was jerked back and down, foot caught in the stirrup, and Kentucky was dragging me on the ground. I must have passed out.

That's the last thing I remember until I woke up in a hospital room and found out my back had been broken. The pain was intolerable until the nurse gave me an injection of morphine and the burning slowly subsided. I woke up the second time in a hospital room and I saw my family around me. I knew something truly terrible had happened. I sensed that my accident had hurt not just myself but also all of those people who loved me. I was told I had just gone through a ten-hour operation to fuse my back together. When I looked at my side I could see stitches that seemed to go on forever. I was told the doctor took my pelvic bone and fused it into the broken part of my back. My back was still broken and an eighth of an inch from my spinal cord. Dr. Brown had just fused it into place without chancing on moving it back. So today I still have a broken back, but encased in a block of my own bone. I thought that Dr. Brown was pretty smart doc who made a pretty smart call.

I stayed in a hospital bed for the next three weeks. Every few hours, the nurse gave me an injection of morphine. Just a few days before leaving the hospital, they took me out of bed for the first time. I could barely walk from the pain and the haze from the drugs. I was going to have to learn how to walk all over again. I started out with a walker and only graduated to a cane much later.

From the outset, I saw drugs as part of my recovery. The day I left the hospital, the doctor wrote me a prescription for Percodan, a very addictive opiate. He even told me that I might want to take a couple for the ride home from the hospital. Some amount of pain is a normal part of recovery from a severe physical injury, but I had come to believe that even slight discomfort was intolerable. I had no idea that I was already addicted to the morphine that they had given me. The regular injections had gotten me hooked.

As my parents, David and I drove back to Ashland, an incredible feeling of terror and panic came over me. I started sweating and my body began to shake. None of us knew it, but I was going through withdrawal from the morphine. We stopped alongside of the road to try to calm me down. Nothing worked, not cold water, not the fresh air, not deep breathing.

The pain came over me with a vengeance, as if my body was being crashed against rocks in a riptide. I panicked. I took one Percodan, waited a while, and took another one. The pain began to subside. That moment was the real tragedy, because my addiction was telling my body and soul that any time there was a problem, there was a drug or drink to help solve it. From that point on, every time I felt discomfort, physical or emotional, I reached for my bottle of pills.

Excruciating pain ruled my life for months to follow. I continued to take my prescribed Percodan. Before you knew it, I was also taking just a little more...half a pill here, a whole pill there to take the edge off. In my gut, I knew that I couldn't take the pills forever and I decided to stop. The medical treatment of pain has come a long way since that time. Back then, no one ever told me about tapering down my dosage. When I decided to stop on my own, I did it cold turkey, without any consultation with my doctors. Obviously, this was not the way to come down off Percodan.

A few days into my self-directed detox, Pam Dixon, my long time friend came by to take me to lunch. Full of willpower, I skipped my last evening and morning dosage. In my friend's car, the sense of dread came over me again. I started to perspire heavily and I was in a full-blown panic attack. My addiction knew what I needed and I snapped at my friend, "I need to go back to the house right away."

I walked into the house and went straight to the medicine cabinet. I took two Percodan. I began to calm down. Within a half an hour, I was back to normal.

Looking back, I see that feeling better after the first few minutes were purely psychological. The medicine hadn't even had time to take effect. I told myself that the pills were for the pain. In reality, the pills had become an emotional security blanket and the pain had become secondary. I was taking medication to quiet my fears about who I was and what direction my life was taking. I realized that the pills curbed my appetite and I was not interested in eating. I was an addict. A long road lay ahead for me. Over the next several years, I switched from one substance to another and ended up drinking and doing Valium daily.

AGAIN, AWAKENED BY THAT familiar feeling of being soaked in a cold sweat, I realize this disease is calling me once more in the lonely dark of night. I find myself sneaking out of bed to take swigs from the pint of Gilbey's gin as if I were drinking gulps of cold lemonade. David standing there watching. "So this is what it has come to, your drinking in the middle of the night?" I was caught. I could see him out of the corner of my eye. "I have this phlegm in my throat and cough that I'm trying to quiet, so I can sleep." He just walks away. I'm thinking, well let's discuss your daily drinking. Yeah, you're the one who can put away inordinate amounts of beer. Here I am, same clothes I had on yesterday that I slept in last night, hair smelling like vomit. I have no real sensations, physical or emotional. I was completely anesthetized and day-by-day I was killing myself. I ask myself, "Is this my bottom?" I know that in a few hours I will be awakened again to feed the monster within that will never, never leave me alone.

I must weigh a mere 98 pounds. I have no appetite. Besides, who wants to eat when they're drinking and pill-popping all day? My skin is a bluish-gray. I didn't feel well and was tired most of the time. My family and friends finally understood the severity of my problem with alcohol and prescription drugs. Keeping a promise to them, I reluctantly went to see a physician friend of mine who I had grown up with. I still remember that conversation, word for word. My doctor friend entered the treatment room with a grim look on his face.

"Your blood work looks pretty bad. You have pancreatitis and I have to admit you to the hospital."

"How did I get that?"

"I suppose from the drinking."

"I barely drink." The denial of this disease is amazing. I was going to die but still I continued to argue with him.

"I smell alcohol on your breath now. When was the last time you had a drink?"

I wanted to lie, but he knew he had me. "Look, I can't sleep sometimes, so I get up in the middle of the night and fix a drink. Last night was one of those nights."

"I don't ever recall seeing you look this way. You know, you're not taking care of yourself."

"In other words, I look like crap." I knew he was right.

"I suppose you'll need to detox so I'm going to refer you to St. Mary's in Huntington. I know a good man there who will take care of you. I'll give him a call."

Still, I wanted to bargain and get out of confronting my addiction head on. "Let me think about this and I'll get back with you."

My friend, the doctor, knew that the time for bargaining had passed. He put the facts as plainly as he could, "We can't let the pancreatitis go, you'll die from it."

I paused. I heard that statement, loud and clear. "Well, let me get home and pack some things."

I left his office and felt like the end of the world had just come. I was scared. No, I was petrified. I had just been ordered to treatment and had been given a lethal diagnosis of pancreatitis all because of alcohol. So what did I do? What any alcoholic would do, I went home and drank everything I had stored in my cabinet. I still showed up at St. Mary's Hospital later that evening very sick and very scared. Still, I tried to think of every reason that treatment wasn't a good idea: I wasn't really an alcoholic. I couldn't take that much time off work. I needed to be with my family. I tried to convince myself I only took pills for pain and anxiety caused by a very serious accident.

I knew that all my anxieties about entering treatment were normal for someone with the disease of addiction. They all point to the real fear, which is giving up the addiction or one's security blanket. After all, in the sick state I was in, I truly believed that my addiction had been my best friend for many years. Only one fact forced me into treatment: I realized that it was either rehab or death and she would make the choice. My pancreas was shot from the alcohol and Valium and, without treatment, I was surely going to kill myself. I also was threatening my family life as well.

The actual admission to the hospital seemed to take forever. A clerk took the insurance information, and then a counselor came to do the intake for admission to the unit. Even though I was a voluntary admission, I fought everyone at every turn. The first thing the counselor asked was for my name. The first thing that I told her was that I refused to be admitted to a locked floor. Her questions seemed like they would never end. She asked for the standard information, name, address, birth date, etc.

She started with the heavier questions: "How much do you drink?" Here I was admitting myself to a rehab program and still I felt the need to lie, "Hardly any at all. I just want to get over this pancreatitis and get off of the pills. I am not an alcoholic. I still want to be able to drink a little. The alcohol was never the problem in the first place. It's the pills. They're the real problem." To my addicted mind, I told a convincing tale.

She never cracked a smile or missed a beat. "So how much do you drink?"

Pushed into a corner, not wanting to give up my drinking, I started with the real lies. "Oh, maybe two or three drinks a week. I'll drink Jack and Coke, especially if I can't sleep. You know, hardly any at all."

I didn't know why, but she didn't press further about my drinking, but instead she moved onto the pills. "How much Valium do you take?"

"I take Valium every day, off and on all day. It just depends on how stressed I am."

At that point, the realization was sinking in about how much I really took, so again I started to cover up the truth of taking Valium all day, every day. I would take three or four of the yellow ones. Sometimes, I couldn't remember how many I really would take, especially if I drank with them and I couldn't tell anybody how insane that was.

The questions continued and got into everything from how many pills I had taken in the past to what kind and for how long. She didn't get back to the alcohol questions and I thought I had gotten away with something until the actual detoxification began.

The detoxification of an alcoholic and/or drug addict is a very specific, scientific process. When I lied about the number of drinks and the number of pills I regularly consumed, little did I realize the pain I was setting myself up for, so, by the third day, I started to experience the DTs (delirium tremens). I went to the nurses' station to demand help. I felt like I had bugs crawling all over my body and I needed a Valium or a drink. Yeah, like they were going to give me a drink. The nurse, indifferent to my complaint and with what I took to be a condescending smile, said, "You can have

Phenagren if you're nauseated or an Ativan." I stuck to my guns and screamed at her, "I don't want those, I want a Valium or a drink and I want it NOW!" Her attitude put me through the roof. She looked up and through her pursed little lips responded, "I'll call the doctor when I get time." My body was raging for the drug. I stared her down and shouted, "I'll rip this nurses' station apart if you don't give me a Valium."

Truth be told, she was never at risk and, despite what I thought, I was never in charge of the situation. Right away, she had pushed the emergency button underneath her desk to summon help. I looked over my shoulder to see two huge men preparing to grab me under my arms and haul me back to bed. They pushed me face down onto the mattress so fast that the last thing I remember was turning to see the same sour-mouthed nurse with a gigantic needle coming toward my butt. When the doctor expressed concern over the fact that I had threatened to rip apart the nurses' station, I responded like the typical smart-mouthed addict. Still refusing responsibility for my tantrum, I replied, "Look, I want some more of that drug you gave me last night." Eventually, I had to come clean with how much I had been drinking so that they could properly monitor my detox process. Things got a little easier after that.

When I say things got easier though, it doesn't mean that things were easy. The hospital gave weekend passes to patients so the treatment team could see how patients handled being sober out in public. My doctors decided to issue me a pass once my pancreatitis had come under control and I'd been off alcohol and Valium for several days. I planned to go out to dinner and a movie with my family. It might sound strange but, at that point, being out in the world sober was a terrifying thing to me. The world just looks different when you're sober because there is so much more to take in. I now think that the bounty of perception is a true blessing. But during the first steps of my recovery, the over-stimulation was a lot to handle.

The movie we chose to see was *Norma Rae.* It was playing in downtown Huntington at the Keith Albee Theater. I had been in the Keith Albee many times as a kid with family and friends from Ashland. Being out of the hospital on pass was wonderful but, in the middle of the show, I had an intense panic attack. Oh, so familiar. I was out in the world without my security blanket woven of alcohol, Valium and Percodan. Everything in my body and my mind told me to sneak off to have a drink or find some pills. I remember a voice running through my head, "I need a drink. I need a pill." However, thanks to having some sober time, I could use the thought-stopping method to respond differently.

I crawled over all the people in my row and shot out to the lobby to splash cold water on my face from the fountain. I stood by the fountain, close to the cold water, for a good quarter of an hour just to make sure that I was going to be all right. Then, I told myself that I had to go back in to finish watching that movie. I knew that if I didn't sandwich myself in with all those people, I'd never get better. I had to overcome my fears and face the crowds. I went back in and finished the show. During *Norma Rae,* I promised myself if I was able to get into recovery from the addiction of alcohol, I would help other alcoholics and addicts to get well, too. Eventually, I made some progress and my doctors and therapists sent me home for good. That first day out was otherworldly. I walked into my house like some movie star with a pair of sunglasses on. I walked through the whole house twice before my aunt told me I needed to take them off and stay awhile. Truth is I didn't think that I was a movie star. I had learned in therapy that there are better ways to shield oneself from the world than by using alcohol or drugs. For me, that meant putting on a pair of shades when too much was going on. To this day, I still put my sunglasses on when I want to shut out some of the stimuli or when my day just gets too hectic.

After treatment, I spent an hour a week for a few years in a therapist's office to ensure my recovery. The most eye-opening therapeutic work, other than the horrible detoxification that I had just experienced, was the family piece. My therapist was older, perhaps in her mid-50s, very tall and slender. Her thick glasses made her look as if she was full of wisdom, and I certainly could use some "thick glasses" wisdom in order to help me make sense of where I had been.

"I've just been released from St. Mary's Hospital for alcohol and Valium addiction. What a ride that was. I can't believe that I allowed myself to get to this place in life. I'm 31 years old and my life has been nowhere." She fired questions at me before I could think about how to respond. I told her I was getting a little irritated with her rapid-fire questions. My irritation was normal for someone who had used alcohol and prescription drugs to control anger. I now had to learn how to deal with the normal emotion of anger as a sober person.

"Cathy, I will need to get a family history from you."

"What does my family have to do with this?"

"Everything," she said.

"Well, great," I said with sarcasm, halfway glad that I had someone else to blame besides me. I thought, typical therapist, going back into the past to show that my mother's coldness or my father's overindulgence caused my alcoholism. I loved it. Her rapid-fire questions started again and I found myself loathing this woman and couldn't wait to get out of her office.

I stopped her about halfway through the questioning and said, "Look, let me just tell you what I know about my family. I find that easier for me than you asking me these questions."

"Well, we're out of time for today so why don't you think about your family history and let's start next time with that issue."

I left her office thinking, "That's why I'm paying her so she'll tell me. I don't want to have to think, and besides, I haven't thought much in the past ten years anyway." My appointment with the therapist was exactly one week later. I entered her office and sat down in the same place as before.

"Well, have you thought about your family history?"

"Yes, and I have to tell you, the past week has been a revelation."

"So, you were told you had 16 deaths within your family that were a direct or indirect result of addiction, and you thought it was just bad behavior?" My therapist asked.

"I know I thought that. I would hear sober family members say that a person should just stop. We thought it was just bad behavior." I started to relax with this woman who only a few weeks ago seemed like a total stranger who expected me to spill my guts to her. Once I opened up, I began to talk about the family secrets I had kept only at the surface of my memory for many years. "A few of these family members have gotten into recovery, my father and me being two of them. But, my brother George was still drinking. It was sad to have to witness his slow suicide by alcohol."

I remember how my parents tried so desperately to fix George. They would help buy him houses, thinking that he would settle down and become more responsible or not drink so much. They once bought a cabin on the Little Sandy River. I remember the dialogue between my parents about how good the cabin would be for George. All along, they were hoping that this last purchase would help him quit drinking. My family's entire focus was around his drinking. I would hear the arguments between them, each blaming the other for his drinking. All along, they simply needed to be educated on the fact that chemical dependency was not their fault.

"You now are starting to get the big picture, Cathy that your alcoholism and drug addiction are genetic and you've probably inherited the gene from both sides of your family. The highest incidence of alcoholism is first in the Native American population and second in those of Scottish and Irish descent. You're loaded genetically." Now it all started to make sense why I couldn't get enough alcohol once I started drinking.

It took several months to get my energy back and to feel halfway human again. I continued daily with what I called my soul food: I prayed and meditated on spiritual readings. I got in touch with who I really am without the booze or the pills. Some of the things in my new life I liked and some I didn't. There were plenty of things that made me angry or scared or just plain set me off and made me want to drink. But, instead of running back to my old ways, I prayed and learned how to accept all aspects of my life. I meditated on the Serenity Prayer daily. What a miracle that such a simple prayer truly has the power to change lives. In case you don't already know it, it's simple to learn:

SERENITY PRAYER

*God grant me the serenity to accept the things I cannot change, the courage to change the things I can, and the wisdom to know the difference.*

REINHOLD NIEBUHR

I had been out of the hospital only a few days when I entered the 12-step program, Alcoholics Anonymous. I remembered my promise of helping others, so the 12th step: Having had a spiritual awakening as a result of these steps so we tried to carry this message to others, and to practice these principles in all our affairs had become my focal point in recovery.

David and I thought one way we could have a fresh start on our marriage was to move to Texas. The morning we were leaving for Texas I went down to see my mother. George visited our mother every day and took her a Snickers candy bar. George looked angry because I was leaving them. I didn't realize until much later how much they depended on me. He looked, as usual, his unkempt self and his lack of hygiene were both quite apparent, which I realize was part of his mental illness. I swear his clothes were the same clothes he had worn for five years. He continued to shave though. His face always looked smooth with signs of aging. I have always wondered what it would be like to have a normal conversation with him. "We're packed and ready to go." "Yep" was all he kept saying over and over. I thought I was seeing the movie *Sling Blade* all over again. I hugged my mother and, as I went over to hug George, I could feel him stiffen up and start the same "Yep" all over again. I'm standing outside my mother's place when he walks out. He doesn't say one word to me as I watch him walk down the sidewalk. I could see in his hip pocket his small half- pint of Early Times bourbon sticking out as he walked away. I watched until he was out of sight.

It was July 1981 when we took off for Texas. We took our time in traveling there by trying to stop at each tourist place on the way. We stopped in Nashville where Diana was living, but couldn't find a phone number for her. I later learned that she lived out in the country and didn't have a phone. When we finally arrived in Texas about a month before school started. The temperature was over a hundred and the heat index even higher. I thought perhaps we had entered hell. I had never been in or lived in a huge city like Dallas/ Fort Worth, where it seemed that every freeway was a crap shoot if you made it out alive or weren't maimed in some way. Between the heat, the crowds and the traffic, I wasn't sure if I was going to make it there. I was newly sober and had moved to a large city where I knew no one, but Tanner. Tanner ended up in a town called Arlington that is situated between Dallas and Fort Worth. I went to see Tanner after being there for only a few days. I told her I didn't know if I could survive there. She said, "What kind of choice do you have Napier?" I knew she was right. I wanted to take my daughter and leave, but to where? I basically had no family, no money, no job, newly sober, and little education. In my rational mind, I knew that all those things were stacked against me. In my rational thinking I knew those are the things that lead to homelessness. I knew that, for at least that day, my daughter and I had a roof over our heads. Also I was newly sober and, knowing that change can be very difficult for a recovering alcoholic, I put together my continued plan for recovery. My first priority was to continue working the 12th step of Alcoholic Anonymous: I wanted to continue giving back. I attended meetings regularly, but was still too unsteady in myself to sponsor anyone. I was still shaky and fragile. At times, it seemed as if my every nerve was exposed. I would break out in a sweat with every new situation I had to confront, especially in meeting new people and having to converse with them. Just the very thought of speaking out in AA terrified me. I must have talked nonstop when I was drinking, but found it difficult without my false courage. My hands still shook from the anxiety of each new situation that I experienced through sober eyes. I knew I wanted to do volunteer work, and I also knew that I had long held a love for Israel and her people. I'm sure that the Federation would have some envelopes I could stuff or address mailings for them, so I called the local Jewish Federation to see how I could contribute.

When a Christian girl from Kentucky calls up the local Jewish Federation, the people on the other end of the line are skeptical and rightfully so. Nonetheless, I was told about Hadassah, a women's organization that supports the Hadassah Medical Organization in Israel. They invited me to an orientation luncheon at the synagogue and I attended. At that luncheon, I met many wonderful women who are my friends today. It was probably obvious that I was the only Gentile in the room. I sat between two lovely people who began to quiz me about my interest in Hadassah. My answer was simple: "I want to support Israel." I certainly didn't go into the fact that I was a raging, recovering alcoholic and needed to give back in order not to drink again. I'd reveal that later and, besides, I knew my heart was in the right place. After a while, people came to accept my commitment as sincere. I attended many Hadassah luncheons and was struck by the consistent preparing of our food and beverages by Max, who was the only male in the room at our luncheons. The fall Hadassah luncheon was held at Congregation Ahavath Sholom in Fort Worth. I hear a voice out of the corner of the room say, "Max, what is this? The coffee is too weak. Is this tea?" I watched Max, always wearing his Yarmulke, not hurrying to try and make more coffee. Max was always intriguing to me because he said very little. I always wondered if preparing Hadassah luncheons was Max's only job. I also wondered why Max never said anything and rarely smiled. One day, I was over getting myself more tuna when Max was close enough for me to see the tattoo of numbers on his arm. I had no idea that Max was a Holocaust survivor. I now understood Max a little bit more and why he probably didn't get too rattled over the small stuff, like coffee tasting like tea. Max, the luncheon was perfect especially the coffee, I said and he finally smiled at me. Many luncheons came and went and Max grew dear to me. He would always make it a point to say hi, not much more than hi, but I knew that Max knew my deep devotion to this cause. There was this deep love between us without ever saying a word to one another.

I was able to work on a mission called Operation Moses, where I raised monies to help with the evacuation of thousands of Ethiopian Jews who were air-lifted out of Ethiopia. I approached a pastor of a local church in Arlington to take up a special offering for this cause. I met with Pastor Hester at the Arlington Christian Center to pitch for the cause. "Will you get the church to donate some money to a Jewish cause that the Jewish Federation is involved in?"

"What sort of cause?"

"Well, I have been asked to not talk about it because it's secret. It could blow the entire operation."

"Let me get this straight, you want me to ask my church to donate to a cause that you can't talk about?"

"Yes, that's right.

I'm asking you to trust me."

"Okay, I'll take up a special offering on Sunday night in addition to our regular offering."

"That's good enough."

He kept his promise and sure enough he took up an offering of several hundred dollars that I was able to deliver to the Federation to help with what later became known as,"Operation Moses." It was wonderful getting updates on the young children, who were called Falashas. The very fact that they were able to not only escape horrible famine, but had the opportunity to become educated with the monies that were raised was indeed a miracle. I worked on many fund-raising campaigns and became a life member of Hadassah. I have to say the hardest work I did was working in the annual Hadassah rummage sale. Erika Hochester called every year for me to help sort clothes and hang up shirts that were donated by Panhandle Slim, the Hochester's western wear business.

My involvement with Hadassah and the Federation was the same year the Judd's had just taken country music by storm. Naomi Judd aka Diana Ellen Judd and Wynonna had just come out with their new hit *Momma He's Crazy.* Tanner called and said, "Have you heard Judd's new song yet?" Tanner and I were excited for her. "Well, Napier do you think she should still stick to nursing?" I had told Tanner when I heard Judd was traveling all across the country with Wy that she should just settle down and stick to nursing. I guess I would eat those words after her big success. Tanner and I were always her biggest cheerleaders.

Tanner called and said that The Judd's were going to be in Dallas so we called Judd's assistant to get tickets. My friend and I sat with Tanner and her boyfriend, who later became her husband. We were given front row seats by Judd and, afterward, Tanner and I went to the parking lot to visit Judd and Wynonna on their bus. Judd was always happy to see us. We always exchanged news from home with Judd.

ON ONE PARTICULAR SUNDAY afternoon, I received a call that would change my life forever. I answered the phone and a voice on the other end said, "Hello this is Cipa Taylor. Am I speaking to Catherine?"

"Yes, this is Catherine."

"I'm calling on behalf of Hadassah. We're raising funds for a special project and we were wondering if you would like to contribute?"

"Of course, I would."

Then, there was a pause. After a few moments, Cipa said, "You're not Jewish."

"No, I'm not Jewish."

Kind but confused, Cipa asked, "Then, why?"

Why? I had met the question before. "I want to support Israel." Usually, my response ended the conversation. Cipa's response was different. She said that she wanted to meet me.

We met later that week at an art show sponsored by Ahavath Shalom. I recognized Cipa the moment she walked through the door: an elderly lady with beautiful white hair and sparkling eyes that seemed to dance as she looked across the room. We knew immediately that we were going to be lifelong friends even though we were generations and worlds apart. Cipa was an 82-year-old daughter of an orthodox rabbi and was raised in New York. I was a 32-year-old Kentucky girl recovering from alcoholism and drug addiction. We both knew that God had brought us together.

Cipa became my mentor. She taught me about Judaism, Israel and the people who I love so dearly. More than that, God used her to keep me on track with practicing the 12th step. That wonderful 82-year-old showed this alcoholic that I did not have to give up on life, but to live and give back. I shared just about everything with her about my life. She shared with me some very intimate details of her life. Our bond was so close that she would refer to me as her late-in-life daughter.

I tried to visit Cipa every Saturday or Friday evening. She was orthodox and observed the Shabbat from Friday sundown to Saturday sundown. We spent many nights sitting in her living room, watching the sun go down and talking deep into the night. Her Shabbat dinner table was a holy place and our time together was a holy time.

At first, it seemed like any other end of the week rush hour. I was speeding from Arlington to Fort Worth, about a 30-minute trip, trying to get to Cipa's before sundown. I had one eye on the sun, one eye on the speedometer and, in between, was trying to keep another eye out for traffic cops. Friday night rush-hour traffic in Dallas/Fort Worth is bad enough when you don't have some place to go. With the winter sun setting so early, I was really feeling the pressure.

The rain was cold and somewhat damp, which was unusual for Texas weather. I could feel the cold seep through my clothes like my body was being packed in ice. My thoughts went to thinking that this would've been a day I could've stayed home by the fireplace, but I knew that Cipa looked forward to these visits as much as I did. I had decided today would be the day to tell her about the horrible problem I've had with alcohol. I couldn't tell her that she'd been a sponsor to me, she probably didn't even know what a sponsor was. Besides, I thought, she has lived such a kosher lifestyle, she may think I'm a bad person. These are the thoughts that my therapist warned me about, the very ones that sabotage recovery. The entry into her apartment was always the same ritual we observed, we greeted with a hug, walked into the living room and sat down without a word almost as if we had been conditioned to do so. We would sit in her living room with no lights and discuss whatever was on our mind.

"Cipa, do you know that I'm in recovery from alcoholism?" The silence that came from that one question was eerie as she had just been given a bit of bad news.

Cipa finally broke the silence. "The Torah says if we help save a life then we are responsible for that life."

"I'm not sure why God has put two of the most unlikely people together as friends, but I know there's already good that has come out of my knowing you."

"I won't let go of you."

"Cipa, I never intended for you to help me. I started calling Hadassah and the Federation in order to help them."

Cipa, through her head back with her mouth wide open and let out this huge laugh. I was puzzled that she was laughing. "Well, isn't that just the way God works," she said. "We both have benefited from your 12th step of Alcoholics Anonymous."

I knew what she meant. I had followed the 12th step of giving back. I knew that the one place and people I love was the place Israel and her people, so that's where I started and ended up having my entire life changed.

It was my birthday and I received a note from Cipa that read:

*Cathy,*

*This note is for the "daughter" of my old age, for her and her family to enjoy for all the good years ahead. We wish you fine health, peace, contentment without end."*

*Cipa and the Cristols*

Cipa called later and invited me over for a birthday dinner. My birthday is in May, so sundown comes much later. I arrived just as the sun was setting. Her living room had become a sanctuary for me. This was where I was able to talk with her about my innermost thoughts. We prayed and, then in the dark, we ate by candlelight.

"I had a craving today."

"What was that like for you?" She had become my substitute therapist, my friend and my confidante. This was never the plan, it just happened. She stepped into the role as a natural. She just allowed me to talk without judging me. I don't think I had opened up to anyone before like I had with her.

"It's something I can't keep secret. I've kept so much secret to the point it has caused me harm, but this desire can't be kept secret. Sometimes I don't want to tell anyone, but I know the consequences if I keep it secret, I'll drink."

"I have something for your birthday," she said. "I hope you get addicted to this." She hands me an uncooked Empire kosher chicken. I looked at it and chuckled.

"A chicken?"

"Rachael laughed too when I asked her to pick up one for your birthday."

I told her, "I'll cook it this weekend for my family."

It was a Saturday afternoon in late spring when the Van Cliburn piano competition was playing at Texas Christian University in Fort Worth, Texas. I traveled to Cipa's where we listened to the competition on her radio. We said nothing the entire time we were listening to the finalist. I was content just being in a room with her. We had become so comfortable around one another that it really didn't matter where we were or what we were doing. Her very presence gave me peace.

I received another note from her, which read:

> *Can life be any richer? Yes, friends like you make each hour of each day a divine gift. Please double your visiting hours. I can't get enough of a good thing! I send you my love, and all my thanks for your devotion and your caring throughout the years. Hail to our friendship that will get even tighter, and even more binding! But will always feel free, and at ease! And I have saved my "final" thanks for that Hadassah certificate to mark my birthday. As you can see, my fingers refuse to be pushed around. So, to save your eyes and mine, I'll yield.*

On one special Friday evening Cipa's words jolted me into action.

I pulled into Cipa's and sprinted to her front door just in time. I walked into the familiar darkness, scented with the aromas of dinner. Cipa took my hand and led me to the menorah. I prayed silently for my family and friends as Cipa lit the candles. When she finished, we stood there in the glow. Cipa's face was smooth. She barely had any wrinkles at all, except when her smile brought out her laugh lines. Then she said, "You must go back to school and prepare to do the work God has called you to do." I believe that God was speaking through her. I didn't say anything. I just listened.

"You said you would like to become a counselor. Go and help others because this is what God would have you do." Then, with her characteristic sense of humor, she snapped, "Well, what's stopping you?"

I just nodded my head. It all hit me: What was stopping me? A sense of peace came over me about having some direction and purpose. All my energy, up to now, had been trying to work a program of recovery, which so far, had been successful. I also knew that at some point the addict has to start living life, which means making plans and setting goals. My gift of spiritual discernment saw God's wisdom and love glowing in Cipa's eyes. The meaning and purpose of my life echoed in her simple words, "Well, what's stopping you?"

My journey to get to know myself sober was something I had been doing since my first week home from treatment. I knew that I was fragile in many ways and the one thing I could never do was get myself into stressful situations. I knew going back to school would be one of those stressful situations, but I took Cipa's advice and enrolled in college.

ASHLAND HAS ALWAYS BEEN a safe haven for me. After some of the tragic events in my life, which included my divorce from David, I went to Ashland for a break. I ran into John Deathridge who told me Tanner had been in town. He said, "You need to talk with her. She needs you, she's in bad shape." I hadn't seen Tanner since she left Arlington after she and her abusive boyfriend suddenly got married and she told me they were moving out of town. When I got back to the Metroplex (the Dallas/Ft. Worth area), I called her old boss, who then gave me Tanner's contact information. He quizzed me and then said, "I'll need to call Mary (Tanner) before I can give you her number." My first thought was HE did it again. I got Tanner's number and gave her a call.

"Tanner, what's going on?" I asked, desperate to know if she was OK.

Tanner started talking and didn't stop for over an hour. She said, "We were having Sunday dinner when I asked a question about a meeting he had went to earlier in the day. He got up from the table and started dragging me by my hair to the floor. He kicked me in my back then pulled me up on the bed and covered my face with a pillow. He held the pillow down until I couldn't breathe. He would lift the pillow long enough to punch me in the face and bite me. He suddenly stopped and went into the utility room to get the vacuum cleaner to clean up the mess that was made from food crumbs that had fallen over the floor. I knew that when he came back he would kill me, so I leaped out of bed, ran out the back bedroom door to the back fence. I climbed the back fence and ran to a neighbor's house to call the police. I ended up in the hospital because he had kicked me so hard in the back that I was peeing blood."

"Tanner, when I get a weekend free I'm coming to Houston to see you."

It seemed liked tragedy was all around me. I would barely recover from one problem when another would come right back on top of it. I couldn't understand why my life was surrounded by addiction and violence, but I supposed there must be a bigger plan in all this much more than my finite brain could understand at this point.

Back in Ashland, the call came in from a worker at the Salvation Army. I was elated because George had not been seen around town or heard from in a few years. I assumed he was dead. I put out a missing person's report on him, but I think the authorities didn't look too hard. Everyone in our little town knew George was the town drunk. They probably thought he was on a long drunk somewhere else in the country.

"This is the Salvation Army. Are you Cathy Napier?"

"Yes."

"Your brother George stayed with us for a few nights and then we had him transferred to King's Daughters hospital. We took a pint of whiskey from him that was half empty and he was starting into DT's, so we had him transferred."

The tiny hospital looked like a small clinic from the distance, as I remembered how big it seemed when I was a kid sneaking through the place just for fun. As I entered the front entrance of King's Daughters Hospital, my heart began to pound as though it would beat right out of my chest. I climbed the stairs to the floor where my brother lay dying and as I entered the long corridor of Kings Daughters Hospital fourth floor a nurse broke the silence.

"Are you prepared for what you're about to see?" she asked.

"No I'm not," I replied. As I entered his room, I looked to see if he was conscious, and he wasn't. I could see his face only because the light through the window cast a dull bluish-grey over the entire room. He looked at peace, perhaps for the first time in his life.

Life had not been so kind to George. He was raised in an alcoholic home. He was a high school drop-out, a Korean War prisoner (POW), and an alcoholic who had lost everything due to his disease and who was now dying of cirrhosis. I had read about cirrhosis and certainly studied it in school, but I had never seen a case until then. Ironically, my first case had to be my brother.

I tried to talk to him and asked him to wake up. His distended stomach appeared to be swollen four or five times its normal size, and his arms and legs looked quite thin. He reminded me of a victim of the Holocaust. I could see my childhood home from the hospital bed window. Huge tears welled up as I remembered all of my family members who were now gone and I realized that my brother would soon be gone. Many times as a child, I would look out my bedroom window and I could see the hospital lights in the distance, but never once did I imagine that I would be looking at my childhood home from the side of my dying brother's hospital bed. I looked back at him with compassion because I knew the struggle it had been for him to try to get sober and he never could. I felt a little guilty because somehow I had managed to stay sober and live a full life of recovery, yet he didn't get to know sobriety.

I was also a very grateful alcoholic because I was not lying in that bed, because I knew that I drank much more heavily than he did before I got into recovery.

Before leaving for Texas, I went to Miller Funeral Home to make funeral arrangements for George. I kept thinking about the last thing he owned: a pint of whiskey and a Salvation Army magazine that the nurse said he was hiding in his coat when he arrived at the hospital. Here I am making funeral arrangements while he lay dying at King's Daughters and that bottle of whiskey that he didn't get to finish was finishing him off. The whiskey outlived him and continued to survive in his body, slowly killing him by liver failure.

I arrived back in Texas only to get a phone call that George had died. Margie surfaced and took over to finish the funeral arrangements. I didn't attend the funeral because I felt that I had done my due diligence with my brother to ensure he had a decent funeral and he would be buried with dignity.

WHAT FOLLOWS IS A note I received from Cipa in March of 1994. Little did I know this was going to be my last note that I would ever receive from Cipa, though I think she knew that the end was near for her. The note was a card from Hadassah, where Cipa had made a contribution in my honor. The card was a standard card that was sent out to those who were being honored with a gift in their name. The card read:

> With this gift Hadassah will advance programs of Cancer therapy, research, prevention and control in Israel to bring solace and hope to all who seek our aid, to open ever-new avenues of medical pioneering for the people of Israel, and together the world, for all mankind.

Cipa wrote a short note as well. She wrote:

*Cathy dear, it was a blessed day when we found each other. You have made my life sweeter and better. I shall always be grateful for your thoughtfulness, your kindness, your unplanned devotion to this old woman. When can you come to the Passover lunch, remember? Hurry, before the matze and fish are gone for this year.*

*Love, Cipa*

That call came in early afternoon. "This is Rachael, mother has died."

What I said in a low quite voice as if I were trying not to state this bad news loudly or so it would not be a reality if I spoke in a quiet tone. I could taste the salt from my tears as they dribbled down my cheeks. I ask myself, how can this be? I just saw her and she was fine. Here was a woman whom I'd known for 12 years. The tears were flowing freely and my heart ached with a deep loss, more than any loss that I'd experienced, even though my entire family had died. Somehow, I seemed to think she may have known that her time on this earth was drawing to a close. I read that note today and well up with tears and yearning for my old friend, who taught me so much about the real meaning of giving back. Somewhere in her last note to me was the urgency to hurry up and come to visit soon. Work and family had taken up some Saturdays, so going over every Saturday was not easy for me. The gift to Hadassah was symbolic gesture of our friendship. The note was her goodbye to me. During the last few phone calls, there was in her voice an urgency to come now and then the note that stated, "Hurry before the matze and fish are gone for this year." Cipa died within a month after she had written the note. Cipa knew that the end was near for her without telling me or anyone else. That was just like Cipa to keep this a secret as she had kept all my secrets. I went to Rachael's to sit Shiva with Cipa's family and friends. My sadness was concealed as we talked about joyous things regarding her life. Cipa's memorial was in Connecticut, where she also went back to college late in life and taught school, built a house and raised her children.

Her teachings to me were from her beloved Judaism on how to help others, speak kindly to all mankind and treat them with dignity and respect even if you don't like them. Don't treat rudeness with rudeness, but with a kind word. Keep mind and body clean from vileness and all forms of wickedness. Knowing her and others in the Fort Worth Jewish community only deepened my love for Israel, which would later grow very solid roots after an incredible spiritual journey I took to Israel. What occurred during my time there only deepened my connection to God and to Israel. The journey reinforced all that I had learned from Cipa's example and what was demonstrated to me in the local Jewish community. What a wonderful mentor to this recovering alcoholic. My visit to Israel was just as Cipa had described it to me as if she had left an imprint of this in my brain. I could hear her voice as she spoke to me in the candlelight of her living room, "One day you'll be able to go there. One day you will feel as I did when I walked on the holy ground. One day you'll fall in love with this holy city." She was right I felt humbled to be in the same place as the God of Abraham, Isaac and Jacob. I felt so insignificant, so small and so religiously inadequate. My prayer, "Lord thank you for the Jews, because I would not be who I am today without their help." The lessons I learned from Cipa are to always do the right thing even if you don't want to. Always love those whom you don't wish to love. Pray for your enemies. Keep your life wholesome, you never know who's watching. Be kind to those who are struggling with life's difficulties. Always give back to society much more than you've taken from it. Always do good works with faith behind them. Never judge another person. Be compassionate when you see others hurt. If you help save a life out of the mucky mire, then you're responsible for that life all the way to the end, which was the case with me. Cipa stayed with me as a friend for 12 years all the way up until her death.

One day, I sincerely hope that each of you reading this book will have or take the opportunity to go on a spiritual pilgrimage of your own, to truly commune with a place that is sacred and holy to you and to interact with it's peoples in the way that I did, which has continued to bring me joy, clarity, and solace throughout my life and my continuing recovery. Cipa's advice and counsel through the years had been planted way down deep in my soul, so it was my time to help lift up another soul from the mucky mire.

I HAVE HAD THE opportunity to work in some of the best psychiatric hospitals in the southwest. My favorite place where I feel some valuable work was done, not only by me, but some great colleagues, is Presbyterian Hospital of Dallas. In the distance, it sits mysteriously among decade-old oak trees where life-and-death issues hang in the balance. It's spring and the lawns are neatly manicured with freshly cut grass surrounded by flowers of every color. The stately old buildings reflect the strength of the professionals behind those walls. I sit on the grounds of Presbyterian Hospital of Dallas only to reflect on the period of time when Sandy Mullen and I discovered the reason our patients were having multiple relapses in our program. We watched, we documented and we discovered that these women were keeping a deadly secret. Professionals have always wondered why rail-thin women continue to have multiple relapses with their disease. The big secret kept by these women is their little helpers, which are drugs and/or alcohol used to sustain the eating disorder. Our daughters, sisters, mothers, friends and, yes, even some of our men friends, are in trouble as evidenced by the current rise in bulimia, anorexia, overeating and drug abuse. We came to realize that the drugs were not just hard drugs, but drugs that are deemed harmless, ones used every day by everyone, including caffeine and herbal teas. My reflections take me back to one particular patient who I had the honor of helping. I will briefly share a story about our time together here. Perhaps it will resonate somehow with you or someone you know:

One afternoon I get a call from a man by the name of Tip McKay (real name).

"I need to talk with you."

I didn't get a hello or any type of cordial conversation, just a type of arrogance that came through the phone loud and clear. I did my usual line of questioning and decided to see him the following afternoon in my office. The next afternoon I see this good-looking and yes, I was right, arrogant young man stroll into my office. He took a seat as far away from me as he could get. I always opened my sessions with, "Tell me what's going on."

"First of all," he said. "I don't want my family involved, this is my thing."

I wasn't used to patients telling me what their treatment plan would look like, but realized this guy was terrified that he was even in my office and this exterior façade was his wall of fear.

"Okay, your family doesn't have to be involved. That's up to you, but your family can be a good support system for you."

"I'm doing this on my own."

Something I had learned along the way in my profession is to not struggle with the patient, so I allowed him to enter into my program. Tip started outpatient with me three evenings a week. He would challenge me on issues and the only thing I knew to do was nice him to death. I allowed him to vent in group and I allowed him to challenge me without firing back at him. I have had this happen before in treatment and my usual statement to the difficult patient was, "If you don't like this, then there's the door," but for some reason I had more patience for him. When Tip finished in

Outpatient, I knew he had only done this because he was in trouble at home with his wife, whom I had never met, but, with as little disclosure I received from Tip, I knew that was the case. I told him the night that he left treatment that I would see him again. I only got in return his signature smile, a cocky grin.

Several months later I got a call from Tip. This time I heard a different voice on the other end of the phone line. His voice had more of a humble tone to it. Tip had been arrested while smoking crack in the back of a van with a group of prostitutes down on Harry Hines in Dallas. Bail was posted and Tip ended up this time in my inpatient program. When I went to visit him in inpatient, I realized that he looked different than he had when he was in treatment a few months ago. This man who always looked like he stepped out of *Esquire* magazine, always impeccably dressed, had lost more weight and looked disheveled. I asked him if he was willing to open up to me this time. He shook his head yes. I gave him a few days to get fed and get some rest before we started our sessions. I really didn't know this patient, which was unusual, because most patients open up immediately and never stop, but not Tip. Our first session was allowing him to tell me his story, which he didn't reveal much of when he was in outpatient, so this time I felt I was getting to know the real Tip.

Tip had moved to Dallas from Oklahoma due to his wife's work. He was a Vietnam veteran who did one tour of duty. He worked a short time in Oklahoma, but hadn't worked since the move to Dallas a few years ago. Tip spent a good deal of time taking care of their young son and did a wonderful job with the responsibility. Tip had smoked pot since his Vietnam days and never really stopped. He later ended up snorting cocaine and graduated to freebasing cocaine. Tip described days that the paranoia was so bad after smoking crack that he would end up on the floor crawling on his belly, military-style like he did when he was in the jungles of Vietnam. The crack made him so crazy that even a visit from a repairman at his neighbors' house would cause him to bend the blinds back and crawl from room to room too afraid to even leave the house. Many days were spent smoking crack and flipping out. When his disease had progressed, he was smoking crack almost every day and going through most of their family savings. He would put himself into dangerous places, travelling to Harry Hines to smoke in crack houses with dealers and prostitutes.

I liked this guy. I liked a lot of my patients, but this guy was special. I knew he had much potential. He just needed to realize he had a lot to give back and it was my turn to be the Cipa to him. Tip agreed to come back to outpatient and all outpatients met with me once a week for an individual session. Tip was ready to listen to a strict aftercare plan. I asked him. "Okay, you ready to carry no money?"

"I'm not used to having no money in my pocket."

"You can carry $5.00 a day. You then will decide what you want to spend it on. You can either buy gas or eat. You can buy cigarettes or eat. You get to choose."

"I don't know if I can do that."

"Well, you've shown you can't be trusted with a pocket full of money. A pocket full of money is a trigger for a coke addict, so we get rid of that particular trigger and work on the others. Your wife will handle all the money and give you $5.00 a day or you'll need to go see another counselor."

"Okay," he said. "Whatever it takes."

"You'll have to go to Cocaine Anonymous daily and get a sponsor. I need you to check in with your family daily and tell them where you are and where you're going."

Tip didn't like the aftercare plan much, but he realized this was his only effort to save his life and his marriage. In one of our sessions, Tip told me he would like to do what I do. Many of my patients had voiced the same desire in the past, so I told him what I had told them. "Okay, you will need to call the state and get all the requirements you'll need for licensure. I know you have a degree from Oklahoma University, so you've met part of the requirements. When you've sat for all the education classes, then call me and I'll let you do your practicum under me." I told everyone this and no one had done it yet. I knew the process for licensure was a difficult task to master even for someone who has been sober for years. I blew it off as another patient who would give up because it was too hard and too long to achieve. Addicts are people who want immediate gratification and something as tedious as more education and working long hours for free was not something addicts wanted to do.

It took Tip almost a year to sit for all the educational requirements, but he did. He showed up on my door step with his letter of agreement to enter into a practicum putting him closer to the internship and then the state exam. I honored my end of the agreement and allowed him to do his practicum under my supervision. His next step was to do an internship for free. He called and was ready to do his internship, so he was again under my supervision. Tip finished his internship and passed his licensing exam. Tip then went to work for me at the facility where I was the program director. Tip became a well-liked and well-respected counselor. Patients adored him and many were counseled into recovery from his gentle guidance. I left the facility for Tip to handle and he became the Facilities Outpatient Coordinator. Today Tip is still working in the field, continuing to give back to those who are where he's been. Tip has been giving back, as of today, for 15 years. I knew that through his process of recovery, I couldn't just let go of him. I needed to give him every bit of hope to hang on to that he could become a good counselor. I knew that I needed to be a mentor to him, much like Cipa was to me.

I HAVE BATTLED THE drug cartel one patient at a time up until now. I was sitting in my office at Presbyterian Hospital one afternoon when I received a call from the Bureau Chief of Human Services under Governor Bill Richardson, asking me to think about coming to Santa Fe, New Mexico to head up the TANF (Temporary Assistance for Needy Families) Program for the Department of Health of New Mexico. She said the program was a two-year contract. I knew of Governor Richardson and had always liked what he stood for as a Democrat. I asked the particulars of the job description and told her I would have to think about it. I did my research regarding New Mexico and New Mexico's drug problem and realized that there was a huge problem there, especially with heroin. A small Northern New Mexico town called Espanola has the highest number of heroin overdoses per capita in the United States. After reading the articles, my interest was piqued due to the challenge of putting treatment facilities right in the heart of where the drug cartels live and do their business. The job consisted of putting together substance abuse treatment facilities throughout the state to serve the women on TANF whose barriers to work were substance abuse and domestic violence. First Lady Barbara Richardson's focus was Domestic Violence, so the work that was to be accomplished there would coincide with her work. The Governor set out from the beginning of taking office to work at changing the social problems that had plagued New Mexico for generations. His goal was to do something about the lack of behavioral healthcare for New Mexicans, which included access to drug treatment facilities. The first complete intensive outpatient drug treatment program was opened in Chimayo with TANF dollars. Chimayo has the highest illegal drug activity per capita in the country. Chimayo is the home of the Mexican Cartel, all of whom have settled around Northern New Mexico to dispense their dope. Chimayo is also where the nation's highest number of heroin overdoses occurs. So it made sense to open our first IOP in Chimayo.

A great deal of discussion and planning went into opening the first drug treatment center ever to be found in Chimayo, New Mexico. Archbishop Michael Sheehan headed up the trek to the John Hyson Center. Greg Keferle, Executive Director of Catholic Charities, Bernadette Casias, Clinical Director of the Chimayo facility, and Julianne Bodner, Clinical Director of Catholic Charities in Santa Fe, and I met to plan the first open house and blessing of the center. We decided to start the day with a procession to begin at the Santuario De Chimayo and end at the John Hyson Center, where drug treatment had already begun. During the two mile trek, I was recalling the day that my friends from Kentucky came to visit me in New Mexico, almost one year ago to the day. We had made a trip to the Santuario to see the religious site. Pam, Sally, Pat, Betsy, Judy, Sandy, Carolyn and I pulled the van we were renting into the parking lot of the Santuario. El Santurario (The Shrine) was built between 1814 and 1816 and the "miraculous" crucifix of Our Lord of Esquipulas was found around 1810. El Santuario has been called the "Lourdes of America." No one seems to know exactly how this came about. However, there are testimonies that the extraordinary has occurred. Fr. Sebastian Alvarez, in his letter to the Episcopal See of Durango, dated November 16, 1813, expressed his feelings of the people coming from afar to seek cures for their ailments and the spreading of the fame of their cures, induced many more faithful to come in pilgrimage. He did not mention any specific fact, but something was there. El Santuario has been a place of worship from the beginning. The Santuario is a place to pray, to be thankful, to think, to ask, to meditate and experience peace of mind as well as of body.

We had no idea what was in store for us that day as we climbed the hill toward the Sanctuary. We milled around, took pictures and then decided we would enter the holy place. As we entered, we, who are always laughing and talking, became quiet. We sat together on the old benches that lined the Sanctuary. As we sat there we started to grab one another by the hand and maintained an attitude of prayer and meditation. I looked around at these wonderful friends, all of whom I had known since childhood. We played as children in Ashland, we played in the same park Judd and I used to walk in. I have known these women since the 50s and 60s. Sally, Judy and I were born in little King's Daughters Hospital within only days apart from one another. These women knew me better than anyone else in the world and I knew they loved me with a sisterly love. Something spiritually wonderful was happening to us as we sat there, holding hands and praying. The spiritual closeness we all felt became so overwhelming that we all started to weep. We sat, holding each other's hands and weeping as if we were all being cleansed or having some type of spiritual awakening within the core of our being. We sat there for what seemed like hours, but in reality for only a few minutes. Slowly, we moved toward the front of the sanctuary to an opening into the room that holds the dirt. The people of Chimayo believe that the dirt has some type of healing properties in it. My friends all made a circle around me as I knelt to the ground and started picking up the dirt with my hands and putting it into a bucket for us, so we could take some with us when we left. As I knelt down to scoop up the dirt, I was asking God to bless my work.

It was one year later that the trek to Chimayo took place in order to dedicate and bless the opening of the state's first drug treatment facility there. The procession was approximately 1.5 miles long on a wonderful clear day with low humidity, which helped make the walk more tolerable. I looked along the side of the road and could see hundreds of used needles covering the ditches. Here we were, opening the first ever Intensive Outpatient Treatment center in the middle of an area of the country's with the highest rates of heroin overdose per capita. The facility had already received threatening calls and death threats if we didn't close. I kept thinking about the opportunity the TANF women would have to learn how to stay drug-free surrounded in a drug-infested area. I believe God blessed the treatment facility the day I knelt on the ground at Chimayo the year before.

By this time, the Judd's had been famous for many years. All the Judd's had done some great giving back with good works and money for causes they believed in, which worked in line with my thinking about ways to raise awareness for TANF and the clinic in Chimayo. Naomi Judd was in Albuquerque to promote her newest book, *Naomi's Breakthrough Guide*. I was picking her up at the downtown Hyatt to drive her to Border's Books on the west side of town. Naomi and I have always been able to pick up where we left off as young kids. She's been an inspiration to me because I know what she has been through and I know Judd didn't quit, even though she went through some tough times. She kept plowing through life, expecting good things to happen and they did. I have watched her give back over and over to some great causes. She goes to Ashland every July 4th and gathers food items that are later distributed to the children throughout Appalachia so they will always have good food to eat. While I was driving Judd to her book signing, I said, "Judd let's do a project together. Will you speak to a group of the women who are or have been addicted to drugs and some of these women are trapped in domestic violence situations with either a boyfriend or a husband?"

I explained to her the details of what we would do and her statement was, "Sounds right up my alley."

Of course, every workplace has it naysayers. The State of New Mexico isn't any different. There were many within State Government who said I wouldn't get any of these women to attend. The project was much too big or it was too hard to coordinate. I didn't listen to any of them, because I knew that these women needed and deserved to have the money spent on them. At one point the Director of Human Services stated she was going to cancel the event. I told her that the Governor was coming and planning to speak. When she heard the news, she quickly reversed her decision. Since it was an event for women, the Governor sent the First Lady, Barbara Richardson, whose main pet project when she became First Lady was to speak out against domestic violence issues. Other speakers who were Lt. Governor Diane Denish, Attorney General Patricia Madrid, and judges who also had an interest in the lives of young women who were drug-addicted and victims of domestic violence.

Just as I leaned over the banister of the convention center to see only a few women trickle in, my thoughts were, "I'm screwed," and I imagined various scenarios that involved me being run out of town, followed by a laughing, jeering crowd. Then I looked at all the doors and I saws dozens of women pouring into the center. I was seeing over 500 women stepping off buses and entering the doors of the convention center. All of these women were bussed in from throughout the state of New Mexico. Some of these women had never been out of their little villages or towns. They filed into the huge dining area of the convention center, only to sit down to beautiful tables draped in white linen. Waiters and waitresses served them a wonderful, hot lunch as they waited for Naomi to speak. You could hear and see the excitement in them as the band played upbeat music and the entire convention center took on an environment of pure joy. I stepped up on stage to introduce Naomi and fought back tears. Here, she and I were together again in Albuquerque, New Mexico. Both of us giving, with much compassion and caring, to a group of women of whom we both had some understanding of where they were in life because we had been there.

Naomi had been on welfare and I was a recovering alcoholic. Naomi started to speak openly about her life while I was thinking back to the summer days she and I spent walking through the park as children in our little hometown of Ashland, Kentucky. Again, I started to well up with tears thinking about our innocent years as children, but with the full knowledge of the difficult times that had made both of us strong women today. I prayed while she was speaking that these women would grab hold of her message of hope. My eyes scanned the crowd to see the impact her story was having on their lives. Naomi stepped down from the stage and walked out among them only to be close and give many of them hugs. Women were crying openly. Her powerful testimony was planting a seed of renewal in their lives. Some of the women were in the substance-abuse intensive outpatient program that I implemented throughout the state. I knew that they were or had been on hard drugs such as methamphetamine, heroin and cocaine.

After Judd and I finished what was considered one of the most successful conferences that the State of New Mexico had funded, we parted with our usual hug and "I'll see you." As I watched Judd walk away with her bodyguard, I thought of how much her life has impacted me.

DURING MY VISIT TO Israel, I breathed in deeply, hoping for a fresh start to get involved in something new. I had a revelation while on my journey. I felt led to stay within the same perimeters of the counseling field, as I always had, but with more of a risk involved in helping people overcome their mental maladies. I thought more of a risk than helping the women of Chimayo who entered a treatment facility in the heart of drug cartel country. On the trip to Israel, I had two revelations that had stemmed out of my many years visiting Cipa. As I was walking through the streets of Jerusalem, I remember a conversation I had with Cipa. I told Cipa that my heart was with young women who have addictions, drug, alcohol and eating-disorder problems, and young women who are slaves to prostitution. I remember telling Cipa that I wanted to reach out to these young lives in some way. Maybe even open a safe house for those caught up in voluntary prostitution or by involuntary enslavement. I know that the sex slave trade, whether voluntary or involuntary, in part stems from childhood abuse and addiction keeps them in it. Many young women prostitute voluntary. In a counseling session, I can help them trace back to bondage of sorts, out of being victimized by rape or incest. I've treated many women who manifested anorexia, bulimia, alcohol or drug addiction because of past violations they had experienced. What I've come to realize is that we're not going to beat any of these social problems, but we can be there to mentor those that have had life knock them down. I only pass on what I've learned from my grandmother, my mother, Cipa, Tanner, Judd and my wonderful childhood friends. All of us have the capacity to lift up at least one individual in our lifetime and help make them whole.

Presbyterian Hospital has some of the best care for women suffering from eating disorders. While working there, Sandy Mullen and I realized that not only do these women with severe eating disorders have an addiction to substances as well, but some have had some horrific sexual violations. We treated a young woman who had been gang-raped while attending a college party and later exhibited anorexia; a young mother who was raped by an intruder in her home while her husband was traveling. We have seen many women who have been sexually abused as children by a family member or family friend and one of the symptoms of abuse can be an eating disorder. There was a patient who came to me through word-of-mouth. She was a topless dancer in the Dallas area. She had gotten my name through the grapevine in the night club industry where I had seen a number of patients who had come to me with drug and alcohol addictions. I will call her name Melissa. Melissa came to me because she had a cocaine and alcohol addiction, which is prevalent in the night club business in any major city such as Dallas. She didn't particularly want to stop her topless dancing, which she admitted would often lead to her prostituting herself, especially if the price was right from some financially well-off business man. She just wanted to stop spending her money on drugs. She told me she made anywhere from one to two thousand dollars a night and that she didn't work every night. Most of her money either went up her nose or in booze or in her high-life living expenses. There wasn't anything ugly about Melissa. It was obvious that she worked out daily and had been blessed when it came to good looks. I usually feel a deep compassion for my patients and the dilemma they find themselves in after years of dabbling in drugs, alcohol, illicit sex, gambling and practicing an eating disorder, but for some reason Melissa had sadness in her that I couldn't quite discern. I decided that if she would allow it I would keep her in therapy for some time, even though she had come for a quick fix. During her initial evaluation, I quickly realized that her exercise program, which she argued was to keep her in the dancing business, was indeed exercise bulimia. I didn't press the exercise issue too much, because I wanted other information. She told me how much cocaine she was using and how much alcohol she was drinking. I knew that I needed to multiply that information by about 3 times in order to get the accurate amount she was doing. Melissa's story is one that I heard over and over throughout my years of doing counseling in the Dallas/Fort Worth area. There's a mission field of Melissa's out there. I knew then that I wanted to be a part of helping these women get off the street or out of the clubs, so an organization was formed as a mission called "Operation Mother Hen." Operation Mother Hen is a group of mothers and grandmothers who organize a mission several times a year to hit the streets of Los Angeles,

Atlanta, Dallas and other large cities where prostitution is prevalent to encourage any woman under the age of 21, or even older women, who wants to leave the streets and come with them where they will be transported to a safe house for rehabilitation.

If I had ever asked for a clearer sign, I couldn't imagine what form it would take other than a phone call I received after returning from my annual trip with my best friends from school. After a raucous weekend, I had only been back in New Mexico a short while when Pam called early one morning. "Have you heard the news?"

"No," I said.

"Tanner died."

The sound of that news was charging through me like a bolt of lighting. I didn't know what to say except that I couldn't believe it. Tanner had so wanted to come to our reunion, but couldn't because she was recovering from the back surgery she had in March. Her death troubled me and I kept playing back the recent conversations we'd had about her leaving Fort Lauderdale and heading back home to be with cousins and friends. Tanner told me she was putting things together to make the move. I was sad because Tanner would've been back home and close to people who loved and cared about her. Tanner had her funeral in Ashland. Judd couldn't make the funeral, but her mother, Polly Judd, went to represent the Judd family.

One week later, I had to travel to Winslow, Arizona. The drive to Winslow is a beautiful drive through Gallup, Window Rock and some really gorgeous Native American land, a drive through land where there's hardly ever a cloud in the sky. Many beautiful huge ravens and eagles fly through that area. I was travelling just before dusk when the sun starts to go down. This is a time of day when the sun shines on the rock turning it red, gold and bronze. I started to weep over Tanner. I allowed myself to grieve her death, so I could get it behind me. I allowed myself to talk to God about Tanner. "I'm going to miss our late night conversations. Take care of her Lord. I know that contagious laugh will ring through Heaven. I know she's with You in Heaven, dancing with her family." I had a vision that Tanner was smiling at the wonderful sight she was seeing. The sight of heaven was beyond her wildest dream. "My dear friend I know you're at peace now. I know you'll have no more hardships. Be at rest my friend and one day I'll see you again."

As I STOKE THE deep and wide, old, stone fireplace, I feel the warmth coming out into the room permeating my body almost as if the stealth heat is giving rise to a peace within my soul. My mind races back to where I've been only to reflect on this journey, in this damp, cold morning. I truly believe I have found within myself the only thing that makes sense in this world, which is to touch the life of another human being and those that have hit their bottom are the very ones best-suited for the job. I had only reached out to the Jewish community in order to stay sober, but look how the process of working that 12th step transformed my life. Just think... if every recovering addict, or, for that matter, anyone would work the 12th step daily, what a different kind of world we would see. I have remained in recovery from alcohol for 34 years only because of giving back to those who are still trying to get free from their bondage. I will finish this life with my best and final 12th step work, Operation Mother Hen.

# Assignment for Chapter Five

## PSALM 42

As the deer longs for streams of water,
so my soul longs for you, O God.
My being thirst for God, the living God.
Where can I go and see the face of God?

## *Quote*

Source of Time and Space Avinu Malkeyinu! From infinity draw down to us The great renewal And attune us to Your intent So that Wisdom, Your daughter Flow into our awareness To awaken us to see ahead So we help instead of harm. May all the devices we make use of be sparing and protecting of Your creation. Help us to set right what we have debased To heal what we have made ill To care for and to restore what we have injured. Bless our Earth, our home and show us all how to care for her So that we might live Your promise given to our fore bears, To live heavenly days Right here on this Earth. May all beings Whom You have fashioned Become aware that it is You Who has given them being. May we realize that You shaped our lives And may each one who breathes Join with others who breathe In the delight of shared knowing That You are the Source of all breath. Assist us in learning how to partner With family, neighbors, and friends. Aid us in dissolving old enmities. May we come to honor, Even in those whom we fear, Your image and form, Your light Dwelling in their hearts. May we soon see the day when Your House will be indeed The House of prayer for all peoples, Named and

celebrated In every tongue and speech. On that day
You will be one And one with all cosmic Life. Amen!

Rabbi Zalman Schachter-Shalomi, World Wisdom Chair, The Naropa Institute, Colorado. Excerpt from *The book Prayers for a Thousand Years*. Edited by Elizabeth Roberts & Elias Amidon; Harper San Francisco: 1999.

*Meditate or reflect on the Psalm or the Rabbi's poem.*

## Commentary

THERE IS NO RECOVERY without putting God in your life. People oftentimes want to try recovery as a lone wolf, but soon find out that the addiction is a powerful disease that only something greater than willpower can overcome. I believe that we have to have a transformation from the inside out in order to get into long-term recovery. There is only one way to achieve this goal and that is to allow God's transforming power in your life along with the 12 Step Program. The program teaches addicts how to live life addiction-free. The 12th step has been the most important step for my recovery because it has enabled me to give back to people who are where I was in life and still could be if I don't work this program daily, taking it one day at a time.

## Questions to Answer

1. Do I use illegal substances? If so, what are they?
2. How do I feel about living without a chemical? Write down your feelings.
3. Write down who and what you will need for a recovery support system.
4. How has my chemical addiction/abuse affected my eating habits?
5. Write down a healthy physical wellness program that you can follow to help maintain your recovery.
6. Call your sponsor and mentors daily, because they will become your lifeline.
7. List ways you feel secure in life.
8. Think and write down a way you can work the 12th step. Only work the 12th step after you've worked the other 11 steps.
9. Write down and keep a list of people you can reach out to on a daily basis.
10. Write down one easy goal you can achieve the first year of sobriety.

SIX

# Sandy's Story: How I Found My Calling in Life

I grew up in rural Pennsylvania in a beautiful valley surrounded by hardwood trees. The family business was timber. Our grandmother lived next door and my aunt and uncle lived across the road. From a young age, books were my friends and I became a voracious reader. I was fascinated by the stories of the outside world and I knew I would need an adventure in my lifetime. I also dreamed of writing.

On the day my co-workers celebrated my sixth birthday at high tea, my dream to write was made public. Cathy (an extrovert) announced to the group, "Sandy and I are writing a book." The introvert in me swallowed hard as I thought, "I don't believe she just said that." At the time, I was still working full-time and didn't know when I would possibly have time to write. A place to write also became important in the process.

A WINDING, GRACEFUL BRIDGE connects the town of Port Isabelle to the island of South Padre, Texas. It was late April and my husband and I went there for a week's vacation. My goal was to write. Our children played on the beaches of South Padre and their sweet spirits swam in the warm waters.

The ocean has always been a scared place to me, enabling me to reach deep into my center. The coming in and the going out of the tide washes over me and renews deep places. I also wrote at the Dallas Arboretum, surrounded by the beauty of nature where the seasons unfolded. Our farm in Pennsylvania provided a summer setting. As I look back at the story I was able to tell years ago, I see myself differently now. I smile at how protected and guarded I was. I also took myself much too seriously. This is where I am in my life now.

I am Sandy and I am a compulsive overeater. The patterns for disordered eating were set in motion in my family of origin. The range of the disorder in my family went from food restricting to overeating.

My mother, a tall beautiful woman, was always proud of her thinness. One day, she announced to me, "I was so thin when I was pregnant with you, people didn't even know I was pregnant!" I remembering wondering if that was good for me. I can't remember her eating many full meals except at holidays. She would nibble as she cooked and then say she wasn't hungry. She would sit at the table with a few bites of food on her plate. She always had her cup of coffee.

My maternal grandmother was dear to me and I remember running to her for hugs. She wrapped me in her arms and I felt her unconditional love. She was soft and firm at the same time and smelled like lavender. When Grams came to visit, her joy in cooking was evident in the aromas in our kitchen. She would make her famous coffee rolls. Another memory, which at the time was disturbing to me even as a child, was of her sitting rocking in her rocking chair with a full chicken on her lap, eating in a trance state. Later, in my disease of compulsive overeating, I would sit with a big bowl of popcorn and eat in a trance state.

Growing up, mealtimes were not a pleasant experience for me. Conversation was not encouraged. We were to eat quietly with our mouths closed. Many times, I was told by father to "stop smacking." I glared back defiantly. To survive the unpleasantness at the meal, I ate quickly, barely tasting the food. As children, my parents required that we drank a glass of milk with the meal. This rule was not up for discussion. I never liked milk. I would wait until the end of the meal, scrunch up my nose and gulp the wretched stuff down. The last glass of milk that I mostly willingly drank was at the end of my pregnancy with my third son. Years later, I suspect that I am lactose intolerant.

Mother, who was a good cook, always served our plates and gave us our portion sizes. She was not only obsessed with her weight but she was also obsessed with keeping me thin. At times, I would say to myself, "I want more. Why can't I have more than you gave me?" If there were leftovers, they were for my brothers because they were growing boys.

I pondered, "Were not girls suppose to be growing too?" I am aware that I wasn't given the chance to eat according to my appetite. I can remember sneaking into the kitchen and cutting a sliver from one of mother's famous pies and then denying the action when I was caught.

My father's mother died when I was 12. I saw drawers and drawers full of gum and candy that had grown stale and had to be thrown out when after her death. I wondered why she hadn't shared those with us, her grandchildren, who lived next door. We visited her often and we rarely had those treats at home. In her basement, her fruit cellar had rows and rows of canned fruits and vegetables that also had to be thrown out. Today, I understand her hoarding came from living through the Great Depression and fearing that there would never be enough. Certainly during the times of the refinery strikes (my father worked there after leaving the family lumber business), we as a family would have appreciated the extra food.

Those were some of the food patterns that were presented to me as a child. They weren't completely off the charts in food dysfunction but what I have become most aware of from reading the literature is the genetic predisposition for our body types and the wiring for eating disorder behaviors. Recent research is able to claim that up to 80 percent of our body build is hard-wired from our gene pool and the research is saying that our brains are wired differently when it comes to food. I can first remember overeating in my teens, when I visited a cousin and her husband. They made huge batches of popcorn and I could eat as much as I wanted! And then I could get up the next morning and finish what I hadn't finished the night before. Today, I know this cousin has/had an eating disorder and I also know her mother, my mother's sister, was bulimic. This information came to me from my favorite 80-something-year-old aunt, talking about her sister. It was near the end of her life and I have no reason not to believe her. At the end of her life, she had a need to share family history that even my mother wasn't aware of.

The over-awareness of food was in my childhood. I learned early to use food as a comfort. As a family, we had women who were excellent cooks. The message was, "Eat up and always finish everything on your plate." The other unspoken rule was, "Don't ever gain weight." When I was young and well into my 20s, the family message worked. I never ascribed to women eating sparsely. With smugness, my attitude was, "I can eat whatever I want and not gain weight." I did not have any empathy for people who were overweight and I certainly couldn't identify with them. I now know overeating activates brain chemistry into the disease process for those with the predisposition for addiction.

I had my first son when I was in my late 20s and my third son when I was 35. My eating patterns were well-monitored when I was pregnant. After the birth of my first son, a friend and went to Weight Watchers. I had not lost 11 pounds of the weight I had gained during my pregnancy. I have great respect for the program and, at the time, it presented a balanced approach to weight management. When the weight didn't come off after the birth of my third son, my overeating was well established. I used food to dull uncomfortable feelings that came up in my marriage. My husband was a psychologist and so he must have had the right perspective. Of course, I now know my perspective is and was as valid as my husband's perspective, no matter what his occupation. I was also the mother of three active, bright boys who were the delight of my life. I was in denial and I didn't allow myself to be aware of the pathology in my eating patterns.

At 43, I returned to work as a nurse in psychiatry. A new world opened up for me that I thrived in. I started taking the information I was learning home and presenting it to my husband. Sadly, he wasn't thrilled with the new me. The positive result was a span of time spent together in marriage therapy.

My God had a sense of humor. Four years after returning to work, I was assigned to work on the psychiatric Eating Disorder unit. Only in hindsight did I become aware of the magnitude of that particular, seemingly random, event in my life. I was about to learn a lot about my particular disordered eating, and a lot of other manifestations of eating disorders, that had progressed into the disease that has afflicted me, compulsive overeating.

Vanity and an ever-increasing weight gain drove me to the OA meeting rooms where I learned that compulsive overeating is a living disease. I had been working with the eating disorder patients for six months. It was a good fit for me right from the start. Patients were attending OA meetings on my instructions and they were coming back with stories of being blessed. I was aware of a feeling of jealousy, but could that be possible? All I knew was that when I got home from work at night, food was my source of comfort. I felt like a hypocrite. I told patients not to use food to mask their feelings and I ended up doing that very thing. Even though I took a nursing refresher course, I felt inadequate. I felt I had lost my nursing skills while I was at home for 14 years with my sons. My marriage was a source of unresolved conflict. At times, I felt my life was out of control and I was dealing with feelings of powerlessness. I would go home from the hospital and work out the feelings of the day with seconds of everything as I cleaned the kitchen, or indulge in a bag of chips or a bowl of buttered popcorn. I would eat into numbness and fall into bed at night. The cycle would begin again the next day. The emotional turmoil was an emptiness that was never filled. The food was used to meditate, only to keep the real issues at bay, which it did but only at the cost of weight gain and an emotional shutdown of my feelings.

I made the decision to attend an OA meeting to find out what all the fuss was about. I was also beginning to think that my relationship with food wasn't entirely normal. My denial system was cracking. I sat in the parking lot that night wondering, "What am I getting myself into?" My pride was working overtime, telling me that I was better than that and I was strong enough to handle it on my own. After all, I was a staff member working on an eating disorder unit. "Get a grip," I told myself. I was reticent walking through the door, but I kept telling myself that I was just there to check the place out for the patients in the program at the hospital. I didn't say anything that night as I sat in the circle of 20 or so women who came in all sizes and shapes. They were talking about their relationships with food but I also heard them talking about how food interfered with their life issues. I knew it was time to get real with myself and start looking at the big picture. The stories these women were sharing were real and I knew I was right where I needed to be. I remember listening to them as they read their literature that ended with "Welcome to OA, welcome home." Those words hit me somewhere deep in my gut, and they had me.

The second week, I asked someone to be my sponsor. This wise lady looked me in the eye and said very calmly, "Here is my phone number. Go home and write down foods you binge on and call me tonight." Nodding my head, I was thinking, "Oh great, what have I gotten myself into?" I assured her I would and I did. I was ready for the craziness with food to stop. This would become my home group for over ten years.

My binge food would be identified (mainly salty, crunchy foods like popcorn and chips). My serving sizes would be identified as a problem, as I usually ate more than my husband. The constant, day and night, obsession with food would be handed over to a Higher Power who I call God. Did I really want my last thought of the day to be what was I going to have for breakfast? After breakfast, did I want to be planning lunch and dinner and, of course, was I going to be able to have what others would call snacks but, for me, many times turned into binges. For over two years I kept a food log, writing down everything I ate during the day. I called my sponsor weekly and saw her at weekly meetings. I worked on the steps, which included doing a fourth and fifth step with my sponsor. I read literature and at some point was willing to lead meetings. At that time, my weight did respond to the discipline of the program.

The food was, of course, only part of the picture. I would soon become aware of character defects in myself. I really didn't know that I had character defects when I started sitting in those rooms. I believe that I was afraid to know that information about myself. I soon would learn that I had a living disease that is bigger than me. The circles made if safe to explore myself without feeling judged. I had to be willing not to be numbed by soothing with food. I explored food messages from my childhood. I came to the reality that now, as an adult, I had to take responsibility for my own messages regarding food.

I often tell patients I work with, "I believe that women who sit in healing circles and tell their stories and listen to the recovery stories of other women heal themselves." I firmly believe in the sanity and wisdom of the OA program. After many years, I walked away from the rooms where I learned so much about myself.

Years later, I would return to 12-step rooms as a member of Al-anon when our son went into treatment for addictions. I am two years into this new journey. It was coming home.

YESTERDAY, I READ THROUGH Cathy's story and, as usual, I had tears in my eyes as I absorbed the wonder of her calling. During the night, I had a powerful dream about the collective unconscious. While in church that morning, the thought came to me that it was time to share my great, or numinous, dream, as Carl Jung would call it. When it happened, I didn't understand but I only knew that the dream was not like any other that I had ever experienced. After a few days, I told my husband, the psychologist. He said at the time not to share the dream, to keep it as my own because it would lose its power in the telling. I have followed his wisdom and have only shared it with one other person. So when the thought came to me to put the dream in our book, I was somewhat taken by surprise.

When I was 35 years old, we moved to Austin, Texas. We started to attend St. Ignatius Church. St. Ignatius, at the time, was heavily committed to the Catholic charismatic movement. On a warm day in May, a hairdresser who had been recommended to me gave me "the talk" about the prayer meeting at St. Ignatius and The Life in the Spirit Series, of which she had been a part. Obviously, she had me as a captive audience. Before I left, she had me promising that I would at least go to the prayer meeting. I went home and told my husband, but I was unable to cajole him into attending. The night, as I entered the church for the prayer meeting, I knew that I had been looking for the energy in that meeting my whole life. I would later know that the energy was that of the Holy Spirit. I was so excited that I was able to convince my husband to go the next week. We also signed up to attend The Life in the Spirit Series.

I was very open to the whole experience, and the week before the laying on of hands to receive the gifts of the Holy Spirit, I had this dream. I was aware of a presence, and a magnificent male voice said, "Sandra, I have called you!" I remember thinking that no one ever calls me by the formal name of Sandra. I saw my figure on the ground and I saw tongues of fire come over my figure. I felt what had to be exaltation and I knew at the time that was exactly what I was feeling. When I awoke, I felt refreshed. It took me a couple of days even to tell my husband, even though it was not unusual for us to share dreams with each other. Several days later, when we were prayed over to receive the Holy Spirit, the thought came to me that this was a formality because I had already received the Spirit. My mentor, who prayed over me, was the other person with whom I had shared the dream. It would be 12 years later for me to know that I had been called to work with those with eating disorders. It also took me that long to admit to myself that I was a compulsive overeater. I have been working in the field now for 21 years and I have no doubt that I have been working right where I was supposed to be, with a population that I intuitively knew so much about.

When Cathy and I talked about updating our co-authored book, *Swinging Door of Addiction*, I shared this story with her. At the time, I was working in the Eating Disorder Program at Presbyterian Hospital of Dallas. During an education class, I casually shared this information with the patients, "I am the mother of three sons. I have no daughters." A patient meekly spoke up and said, "But you do have daughters. You have us!" Accepting her insightful feedback, I have had hundreds of daughters. I have given my life's energy to these daughters, walking beside them as they fight the deadly diseases of eating disorders/chemical dependency. I am aware that I have entered the early wintertime of my life cycle. As Cathy and I talked about the update, the thought kept coming to me, "What did I most want to share with my daughters?"

I want to share what I have been writing about for three summers. I have been writing about the relationship between mothers and daughters. I didn't realize until I had written for some time that I was writing about my relationship with my mother as it unfolded before me more and more as I wrote each summer. I have been writing what I am learning about myself as my mother's daughter and what I am learning about myself as the roles reverse and my mother has become childlike and I am parenting her.

We are recovery storytellers and so, yes, Cathy and I will use our ongoing stories in our update. We ask women to continue to be storytellers as they write about their life journey in recovery. We still encourage young women to go to healthy 12-step groups to hear other women who are in recovery for their eating disorders/chemical dependency. I encourage you to listen to how your story is like these women's stories instead of how different or terminally unique your story may be.

In our update, as we start to explore new layers of recovery, we invite you, the women who suffer from eating disorders/chemical dependency, and your families, to join us on this journey by finding your voices and becoming storytellers for the women who will, sadly but inevitably, follow you.

I can trace four generations of eating disorders, as well as alcoholism, in my family tree. Cathy's family can trace the devastation caused by alcoholism and drug abuse. So, our experience is not only as professionals, but as women who struggle as you do. I now want to change hats and tell my story from the perspective of being the daughter of an anorexic mother. This was my first summer of writing. This is my ongoing learning experience of who I am and how I got here.

WE ARRIVED IN PENNSYLVANIA Sunday afternoon after the long drive from Texas. Usually, we spent the first night with my mother, who would make chicken and dumplings and one of her famous pies. The next day, we went to our farm and began the process of opening it for the summer. This includes turning on the water (hopefully this includes hot!), getting the toilets to work, uncovering the furniture, and cleaning the house from top to bottom. This year, we didn't go to Mother's for the night because we had sore throats and cold symptoms that we didn't want to pass on. We met her briefly in the parking lot of a local grocery store and she gave us the ritual food supply she had been collecting for several weeks. At 86, she still lived in the house that I remember my parents building sixty 60 years before. My brother, who lives several miles away, checked on her in the morning and at night.

On a Friday, my brother left a message on our cell phones, "Would you mind going out to check on Mother? She is pretty confused. This is more up your alley. I did fix her breakfast and sat with her while she ate." I called my brother back and assured him we would check on Mother in the afternoon. We suspected she hadn't been eating for weeks and had been living on black coffee. Her cognition had been affected and, at times, she couldn't recall the names of her children. From working in the mental health field for over 20 years, I now knew my mother had been anorexic for as long as I could remember. As a child, I didn't know what that meant. Recently, many of our phone calls from Texas were about her not eating because she didn't like most foods and (especially) she didn't like meat. She said she wasn't hungry and food didn't appeal to her. She said she wasn't able to chew because of problems with her implants. She had, for many years, not attended family celebrations, even refusing the yearly Mother's Day meal at the country club where my brother takes the family. She said she would be too nervous to eat.

My husband and I drove up the driveway and parked the Jeep by the house. By this time, Mother would always rush out the back door to greet us saying, "Where have you been? I have been waiting for you and the food is ready." There was no greeting, only an eerily silent space as I walked onto the back porch. For the first time in my memory, the back door was locked. I knocked and, after a while, Mother came shuffling to the door, still dressed in her bathrobe in the middle of the day. Her greeting was muted; and when I asked her about my brother being there earlier, she replied, "No, he hasn't been here." I decided quickly that she needed to go to the hospital to be evaluated. I said, "Mother, you aren't eating. You aren't sleeping and your words aren't making sense so we are taking you to the emergency room to have someone evaluate you." She nodded in agreement and I packed a suitcase for her. She couldn't tell me where she kept her toothbrush. I easily fell into the task- oriented, charge nurse role. We loaded her into the Jeep and I wondered if this would be the last night she would spend in her home.

Mother was admitted to the ICU for several days and then to a regular floor. It was established she had a right temporal stroke that left her with no physical damage, but instead left her confused and disoriented. At times, she didn't recognize family members. She did start to eat everything put in front of her. Perhaps from the stroke, she forgot the long list of foods that she didn't eat, including meat of any kind. In the weeks leading up to the stroke, she had impaired memory from lack of nutrition. Now, it was impossible to tease out the damage from the disease of anorexia or damage from the stroke or, possibly, age-related dementia. During her starvation phase, she remembered the long list of food she didn't/couldn't eat.

She also had a much-touted list of foods that she was allergic to, and a much shorter list was food she allowed herself to eat.

During her hospital stay, she didn't complain once that she couldn't eat because of her implants. Her allergies were also on hold. She ate whatever was put in front of her. Whenever we visited, she asked, "Have you eaten yet? The staff will get you something." The day Mother was discharged from the hospital, she searched the unit looking for a special meat to make homemade soup for the staff. At one point, she insisted, "Check the hospital ovens to see if the meat is done."

The family decided that she could no longer live alone and chose a Personal Care Home for her. Mother was always a strong, independent, opinionated woman. She was also religious and smart. Her social skills and wit could entertain the masses. I have been told by several relatives she was very beautiful when she was young. In the past, very few care settings could have lived up to her standards; but this time she was willing to try it out."

Mother's adjustment was admirable. She learned to use her walker. She has balked at being told what to do and she was miffed when asked, "Where do you think you are going?" as she headed for the front door that first night looking for her stew meat to make soup for everyone. On one early visit, my husband heard her tell the goldfish, "Now, I am going out to find the meat but you will be OK until I get back." Her search for the meat went on for several days and she was only satisfied when I said, "Mother, I went to your house and I have the meat in my freezer at the farm." On many days when we visited, she wanted to know if we have eaten and could the home provide meals for us. Her preoccupation with food is pervasive. Thank goodness she still eats everything and wants to know when the next meal will be served. She was raving the other day about how good sausage tasted and then said she hadn't allowed herself to eat it for 30 years.

Three weeks into her stay, some of her negativity has come back, along with less confusion. It appears that she was making a case for dismissal from the home because of the way she was being treated. She had an episode when she was given a half of a cup of coffee at breakfast and she demanded more. When my brother inquired, the staff explained residents were given a half of a cup when they started the meal and half of a cup when they finished. That would be especially important with Mother, who lived on black coffee. She also had an incident at breakfast when one of the residents spilled her water and it landed on Mother's chair. She assured staff she was OK but then fumed because her pants were wet. She did get them changed at the end of the meal. She also requested to have her table seating changed. Events such as this increasingly occurred and many times, during daily visits with her, she revealed more stories of her fixed delusions, including people visiting her in the night. We all realized something greater was happening that needed to be addressed.

The family agreed it was time for some anti-psychotic medication to come aboard. I had been requesting them since her release from the hospital. Her doctor was conservative but did agree to them the day Mother was especially nasty to the workers. He ordered a small dose at bedtime, which helped her sleep, and a dose in the morning, which helped her disposition. The day after she started the meds, I was able to have a conversation with her. At the end of the visit, she became tired and the confusion returned.

Before the meds, Mother was pushing to go back to her home for a day or two to see how she would do. "Mother you can't be alone in your house."

She would say, "Oh I know. I will only be there for a couple of days. Do you know where my car keys are?"

"Mother, you can't drive your car now."

She would answer, "I know I can't drive. Where is my car parked?"

The meds did dull the desire to find her car and go home. One day, I brought her to the farm to show her the work being done on the house and to serve her the family soup, the soup she wanted to serve the staff and the family. She approved of the porch being redone in old barn boards and she said, "The soup is good. You are now the official family soup maker." It was bitter-sweet to hear. After lunch, I sat her in a wingback chair with heat on her neck and wrapped her in one of her blankets to take a nap before going back to the home. After much chatter, she finally closed her eyes. I looked at her for a long time, this woman who told me, when I was at the vulnerable stage of puberty, how Hollywood stars would eat so little and get so thin that they would actually starve themselves to death. I learned that being thin was a good thing to do in my mother's eyes. She was always so proud of her thinness. I looked at the woman who judged people on their fatness, at the woman who always told me how much someone weighed and how they had "let themselves go."

I had come to Pennsylvania with unfinished business with this woman, but the life journey of growing older had become the equalizer. At that moment, I looked with kindness on this woman with her great grit and strength. I realized the power the disease of anorexia has had on her life. She must have had resilient genes that have compensated for her abuse of her body. I also saw her physical beauty, still present at 86.

"Mother, when I was young, I wish you had told me stories about inner beauty and spiritual growth rather that about physical beauty. I wish you had been focused on your inner beauty and shared your spiritual journey with me rather than being obsessed with your physical appearance. I always knew about your inner beauty and that is what I loved about you."

Mother has been at the personal care home for three months. For the staff, who cares for her daily needs, it must seem much longer. She is a difficult woman to please and I find myself talking to her often about gratitude, a word that has no personal meaning to her. Her car has been sold, which was difficult for her. After a while, she was able to say, "I didn't like that car anyway." Her home is shut down until spring, when it will be sold. She has announced, "I just want to go home for a few days at Christmas."

My mother is not going gently into the night. She has chosen a path of non-stop complaining about her numerous physical maladies, which are hard to evaluate. She has worn her foot in a protective boot for over three years because of severe osteoporosis, resulting in multiple breaks and tears. She has become dependent on the attention she affords the boot. She is always too cold. She doesn't have body fat. In the middle of summer, she would wear three or four layers of clothing and still complain. This woman who was an elegant dresser now looks like a bag lady. However, Mother is discovering the joy of eating and I smile inwardly as she tells me how delicious a certain dish has been, even meat. She asks the staff for recipes, reassuring them she will try the dish when she is able to go home. The personal care home has an open door policy and, as a family, we are pleased with our mother's care. We aren't always pleased with our Mother's attitude. On one of her grumpy days, the office manager framed mother's state of mind very sweetly, "Your mother just has a complaining spirit."

We have been back in Texas a little over a month. I call Mother almost every day. Last week, she told me about a dream she had the night before. She was in her bed at home, sleeping, when her mother came to visit. My mother asked her mother, "What are you doing here?"

Grandma said, "I am going to be with you and spend the night with you."

Mother said she had the most wonderful sleep and she awoke very refreshed.

I asked, "How did Grandma look?"

Mother said, "She looked wonderful. Her skin was so soft and beautiful and she wasn't big and heavy anymore."

The next day I talked to her and she said Grandma had come again in a dream. Mother asked her, "What are you doing here?"

Grandma answered, "You were hurt when you fell. I will spend the night with you."

When I heard the second dream, I suggested Grandma and Mother's sister were coming to get her.

My mother roared, "I am not ready to go yet!"

I said, "It must be comforting to have them come for you. When I get ready to die, I want Grandma, Aunt Chubby and you to come for me."

Mother retorted, "Boy, I will be really mad if they come and I'm not ready to go."

I do think it is beneficial for us to be able to talk about life and death and to acknowledge the next part of mother's journey, a journey that we all get to take. I am so thankful for the summer we had together and the time we spent in each other's presence. Our roles have reversed and Mother has become the petulant child. As we related over the summer, I used the healing power of humor to talk about life and living life on life's terms. It was wonderful because she was able to laugh at her behavior in her current circumstances and we were able to laugh together. In my busy life of raising my three sons, having a career and living far away in the great state of Texas, our relationship had been on auto-pilot for many years. In this blessed summer, with the gift of time together, our relationship came full circle into the healing circle of life. I, the daughter of addiction, will continue to recover from this generational disease.

Please feel free to email us at OperationDaughtersAddicted@hotmail.com.

# ASSIGNMENT FOR CHAPTER SIX

## PSALM 139:13

You formed my inmost being;
You knit me in my mother's womb.
I praise you, so wonderfully you made me;
Wonderful are your works!

## *Quote*

One is not born a woman, one becomes one.

Simone de Beauvoir, The Second Sex

## Commentary

A PHRASE THAT I often have used with the patients is, "What can you take to the bank for yourself?" Now, I will share some pearls from living life on life's terms that I have taken to the bank for myself:

Walk on Mother Earth. Your roots must go deep into fertile soil to survive the cycles of life. Walk straight and tall. Look toward the sky. Be near water. Go to the ocean and be reverent. Be centered and use your intuition. Be still and value silence and aloneness only to hear the voice of God. Be with people who treat you with dignity and respect. Be able to laugh. Know your own value and worth. Love the person today that you are becoming. Affirm and value your physical appearance. Honor your body daily with kindness. Find and follow your passion in life. Work always on humility. Thrive and be a mentor to the women who are behind you.

We have described our stories with honesty but couldn't have told these stories without the tools to help us along the way. The next chapter will benefit you in your day-to-day recovery process, providing you with tools to stay alcohol, drug, and eating disorder free, "just one day at a time."

## Questions to Answer

1. When I think about giving up my eating disorder and chemical abuse, I______.
2. When I think about being healthy and normal, I_________.
3. I would describe my Higher Power in the following way:____.
4. My relationship with my Higher Power is_______.
5. A recent blessing I received from my Higher Power is_______.
6. What am I feeling when I'm bingeing?
7. How can I express my feelings without stuffing them with food?
8. List things that make me angry.
9. What are people, places and things that make me feel insecure?
10. A blessing I have recently given to someone else is_______

SEVEN

# Tools for Recovery

**CHAPTER OBJECTIVES**

✓ *You will learn how to use tools daily for your recovery.*

✓ *You will learn your most powerful tool is your mind and its ability to create images for your long-term recovery.*

✓ *Negative/Positive Imaging*

Getting sober and into recovery has been an ongoing process for me, Cathy. The weeks that I spent in inpatient treatment were only a fraction of the beginning of a new, transformed life. The steps that I used daily for the past 29 years have been the real meat of staying sober and drug-free. I got right into Alcoholics Anonymous and attended daily. It was difficult for me to read because it had been years since I had picked up a book or an article of any kind. Alcohol and drugs won't allow you to read or comprehend, so trying to wade through the 12 Steps was a difficult task. I knew that somewhere in the "Big Book" was a key to sober living. At least, that's what I was hearing in AA meetings.

AA was wonderful, but I needed something more to help me stay sober and drug-free, so I started to organize my thoughts into positive and negative thoughts or images. I would pick several positive images that made me feel good and that would help me to focus on the day or even, perhaps, the future. I tried to be realistic about the goals I set for myself. Then I would choose one or two negative images that would definitely become a reality if I went back to my addiction. I used the negative image when the thought to take a drink would come up. I later called the process The Negative/ Positive Imaging Technique, which I wrote for my own recovery process. I have since used this technique with hundreds of patients to help them achieve recovery.

Simply take a piece of paper and answer the following questions:

## POSITIVE IMAGING

1. What are your personal goals?
2. What are your relationship goals?
3. What are your physical goals?
4. What are your financial goals?
5. What are your career goals?
6. What are your social goals?
7. Who or what is your Higher Power?
8. What do you believe is your purpose in life?
9. Who is the most important person in your life?
10. What's the most important thing in your life?

After answering these questions, decide what positive image would best fit with your future goals. Then, ask yourself what the most important question is. For example, if having a career or higher education is the most important positive thing that can happen in your life, and alcohol, drugs and/or an eating disorder have kept you from maintaining a career or reaching your full potential, then create an image that would put you into the college of your choice, and imagine being in the classroom or walking the campus. If alcohol, drugs and/ or an eating disorder have robbed you of your family life, or if you have lost good friends due to practicing your addiction, then create a positive image that would have you taking a vacation with the loved ones in your life. Actually plan the vacation in detail. Use these images throughout the day, as often as you want, in order to lock them into your mind.

Remember Jesse? Jesse used his young son to help him with his day-by-day recovery. Jesse would picture the smile on his young son's face when he realized that his father was not drinking. He also thought daily about how his son used to avoid him when he was drinking, but now greets him as soon as he walks through the door at home. Jesse said he carries that image with him daily. Jesse's big craving comes right after he gets off work. He wants to drive to the beer store, so he begins thinking about the young boy waiting for him to come home. Jesse also has a picture of his boy over the sun visor in his truck.

## NEGATIVE IMAGING

1. What are the events surrounding your need to seek treatment for drugs, alcohol and/or an eating disorder?
2. What was your drug or destructive behavior of choice; e.g., alcohol, cocaine, methamphetamine, marijuana, bulimia, anorexia and/or compulsive overeating?
3. Are you afraid of death?
4. Are you afraid of a debilitating disease?

5. What are your fears? List as many as you can.
6. What kind of legacy do you want to leave behind after your death?

Again, I'm going to use an example of an image Jesse created. Remember that Jesse said he wanted to break the alcoholic cycle in his family? His negative image was picturing his distended stomach and death as a result of liver failure. He could picture that little boy walking around in front of his coffin, knowing that alcohol had taken his daddy away. This image was very real for Jesse because he had witnessed the death of his own father as a result of alcohol.

Remember Amanda? Amanda used Doug, her husband, as a positive image to keep her eating-disorder- and drug-free. She would imagine the time she and Doug first met and how wonderful the times were together. She would plan out how she was going to regain his trust and have a rebirth of their marriage. She would play the positive scenario over and over in her mind. On one of her visits back to the unit for aftercare, she described their newfound interest in each other. She also knew that just one slip up with the eating disorder or with drugs would have the relationship back into total destruction. Amanda stated that her negative image was imaging the deterioration her physical health had taken as result of the dual addictions. She literally imagined herself barely able to live life to its fullest because of damage to her heart. She realized that the bingeing, purging and methamphetamine usage had already compromised her health. She knew that if she relapsed, the damage could get worse.

After answering these questions, decide which one is the most important to you. For example, if you're afraid of a debilitating disease, then create an image that would have you in a wheelchair or not allow you to exercise, which is quite possible if the eating disorder has damaged your heart or the cocaine addiction precipitated a heart attack. The bulimic could picture having a blood vessel burst in the esophagus and not having enough time to get emergency room care.

Imagine these situations daily, several times a day, implant them in the mind so that you can automatically and effortlessly recall them when the urge to use, drink or practice the eating disorder arrives. Remember that unless you stay drug-, alcohol-, and/or eating-disorder-free, you will never be able to accomplish any of the goals you listed during positive imaging. Relapse will only make the negative images come true, especially the question about being afraid of death. I always ask my patients to imagine seeing themselves lying in a coffin with their family and friends walking by and knowing that the alcohol, drugs and/or an eating disorder have won.

One of my vivid negative images is seeing my brother always with a pint of Early Times bourbon in his hip pocket. I then switch to seeing him lying in the hospital bed with a distended stomach as the result of cirrhosis.

## HALT

That day that I, Sandy, entered the recovery room of OA, I really didn't know what to expect. Over many years, I attended hundreds of meetings. Slogans are used as nuggets of truth. One of the slogans is to "suit up and show up." Even if you don't want to be there, go to a meeting. I do know that you can discover what life issues are struggles for you. I also know that there is grace in those rooms that comes with complete acceptance. It was an awareness to hear others talk about their character defects and to be able to admit that I have the same ones. I could identify the defect, talk about it, and not be judged. I appreciated the meetings being solution oriented once a problem was identified. Before I started going to meetings, I had always believed that others were going to have to change in order for my life to be better, and let me tell you about their character defects. Folks, this is an inside job, and nobody but me has to change for me to be in recovery for my eating disorder.

I do not claim to have new answers for compulsive overeating, but only old wisdom that this storyteller will share about her journey. Eating less and exercising more is still the gold standard in the field. One of the revered 12 Step concepts is the acronym HALT. It stands for hungry, angry, lonely, and tired. This is what HALT has come to mean for me personally.

Hungry represents the first letter in HALT. As a compulsive overeater, it is not an option for me to be too hungry. I must eat three meals a day and have a snack before bedtime. I don't skip meals or fast or use liquid diets. It just doesn't work for me. The compulsive overeating syndrome is always waiting for me to follow that path right into disaster. What does work better is to plan my meals and make decisions beforehand on what my meal will look like. I do eat the five recommended servings of fruits and vegetables daily. I eat protein and fat in my meals. I eat a yogurt daily, and I have a dessert at least once a week. For the first three years into the program, I wrote everything in a food log. It did help to see my food intake in print. If I also felt sorry for myself thinking that I was eating like a bird, albeit a 400 pound bird, I had a reality check. I do not eat below 1200 calories.

One of my very vulnerable areas is serving sizes. I grew up with brothers and male cousins and sons, not post-menopausal women. This has turned out to be a really unwelcome challenge that I can't remember signing up for. I am in the midst of that learning curve. I do know that I will use balance and moderation to the best of my ability on a daily basis.

Angry represents the second letter in HALT. I do not have the luxury to have unrecognized and unexpressed anger. If there is one thing that I have eaten over and over in my life, it is anger. When

I started OA, I did not know that I was angry. From my childhood, I had reasons to be angry. It was my style not to address it because I didn't recognize it. In the first ten years of my marriage, my husband and I did not fight. I did have occasions that I wanted to have a fight, but my husband would not fight with me. At the time, I thought that there was something wrong with me. Years later, I would recognize that my husband is not good at expressing anger either, so it just went on and festered between us. When I went back to work as a psychiatric nurse and then started OA four years later, my denial system was no longer useful or adaptive. Soon, my husband and I went to a couple of years of marriage counseling. Anger is a daily area to check out for unrecognized and therefore unexpressed feelings.

Lonely represents the third letter in HALT. As I have shared earlier in the book, I felt lonely growing up in a family that I didn't feel I fit into very well. I flourished in school, and I was one of the few who really loved school, including high school. I am by temperament an introvert and I renew myself by listening to my inner world. I remember being in the Peace Corps in Iran in the late 1970s and going with all the other volunteers to different places and not seeing an American or speaking English for a week. I had a certain peace about that time that fits my personality. That strength is also a weakness if I don't tell people in my life what is going on with me, they have no clue there's a problem. I must also share what is going on with food when I am having a struggle. That is what having a sponsor serves. At times, I can get so caught up in work and other parts of my life that I lose sight of sharing myself. My husband has also been there to hear me and to listen and validate my feelings.

Tired represents the fourth letter in HALT. I really do not do well without eight hours of sleep. As a teenager, I was a wonderful sleeper and could easily sleep until noon when I was visiting relatives in the summer. At home, one was not expected to sleep very late and so no one did. As a young mother, being sleep-deprived comes with the territory. I really was more aware of sleep when I later went back to work. The job was demanding and I went home to three active sons. Housework was easy to defer to another place and time. In fact, it is still in the deferred category. I have used food to eat my way into energy and it works temporarily. The long-term result of this behavior is a disease.

I have said that I slept like a baby until I hit menopause. The wakefulness and other symptoms of menopause were wearing on me. To be wide eyed at three o'clock in the morning, knowing that I had to get up and go to work in three hours, was frightening. By choice, I have been off any hormone therapy for over five years. I am really glad I made that decision even before the data about the negative consequences was known. I make every effort to get eight hours of sleep, as that is where I function best.

Here are some closing thoughts to share. I tell patients that they can always go back to practicing their eating disorder if they don't like recovery and the gifts of recovery. Their disease will be waiting for them, no questions asked. A useful technique is to have thought-blocking messages to interrupt the shame messages. An example of a thought-blocking message would be, "I am a precious child of God." What would your day look like if you repeated this message to yourself a hundred times a day? Give solid recovery a year of your life. Make a gratitude list of the blessings of your new life. Enjoy the freedom to live fully, with passion and purpose in the gift of serenity.

## Assignment for Chapter Seven

### PSALM 119:50

This is my comfort in affliction,
your promise that gives me life.

## *Quote*

My God, I have no idea where I am going. I do not see the road ahead of me. I cannot know for certain where it will end. Nor so I really know myself, and the fact that I think that I am following your will does not mean that I am actually doing so. But I believe that the desire to please you does in fact please you. And I hope I have that desire in all that I am doing. I hope that I will never do anything apart from that desire. And I know that if I do this you will lead me by the right road though I may know nothing about it. Therefore will I trust you always though I may seem to be lost and in the shadow of death. I will not fear, for you are ever with me, and you will never leave me to face my perils alone.

Thomas Merton, Abbey of Gethsemani, Thoughts in Solitude

*Meditate or reflect on the Psalm or Merton's Thoughts in Solitude*

## Commentary

Following are blessings in recovery that we have experienced in our lives:

1. To be aware of and to embrace your place in the universe
2. To recognize yourself as a child of God
3. To experience the joys and suffering in life with feelings
4. To be in honest and caring relationships with people of your choosing
5. To be able to laugh and to see the humor in your addiction insanity
6. To be used by God to plant the seeds of hope in recovery that touches others' lives
7. To grow old gracefully and with great courage

## Questions to Answer

1. How have I kept the hunger pangs away?
2. Have I used substances to help with the hunger pangs?
3. Do I eat three meals a day?
4. Do I eat a variety of foods?
5. What is the origin of my anger?
6. What are the things that make me angry? List them all.
7. Do I deal with my anger in a positive way or a negative way?
8. How can I deal with my anger in a positive way?
9. Have I incorporated a support system to help me get into recovery?
10. Who is my support system? List them all.
11. Do I get enough rest?
12. What are the stressors in my life?
13. Do I say "no" to requests that will tire me?
14. Have I eliminated the stress in my life? If yes, please list.
15. Have I protected myself from those who don't make me feel good about me? Please list. Think about downsizing your friends who aren't good for you.
16. Do I have healthy people in my life? If so, please list.

EIGHT

# Storytellers

*Our time together* is coming to an end for this part of the journey. We have written about our belief that women who suffer from the serious addictions of eating disorders and alcohol and drug abuse are best treated by a simultaneous, integrated program. Our best teachers appeared when we realized that we needed to listen to our patients and our invitation to you is to start listening to your true self. Issues that you work on while still using an eating disorder or drugs and alcohol to numb yourself will still be there waiting for you to be clean and sober. Clean and sober can best be done in a program that is knowledgeable about treating addictions in a simultaneous, integrated treatment approach. If you do not have access to such a program, find a therapist who will work with you and who has expertise with addictions. Twelve Step meetings will also be a resource for you. Alcoholics Anonymous and Overeaters Anonymous meetings always have people relating their stories of addiction and recovery. The stories are a source of inspiration to every addict. You will also have the opportunity to work the 12 Steps of recovery. Remember, recovery starts from the inside and projects outward. Here are the

12 Steps that we follow that we hope you will incorporate into your story:

1. We admitted that we are powerless over alcohol/ drugs and/or an eating disorder and that our lives had become unmanageable.
2. We came to believe that a power greater than ourselves could restore us to sanity.
3. We made a decision to turn our will and our lives over to the care of God as we understand Him.
4. We made a searching and fearless moral inventory of ourselves.
5. We admitted to God, to ourselves, and to another human beings the exact nature of our wrongs.
6. We were entirely ready to have our God remove all these defects of character.
7. We humbly asked Him to remove our shortcomings.
8. We made a list of all persons we had harmed, and became willing to make amends to them all.
9. We made direct amends to such people wherever possible, except when to do so would injure them or others.
10. We continue to take personal inventory, and when we are wrong, promptly admit it.
11. We sought through prayer and meditation to improve our conscious contact with God, as we understood Him, praying only for knowledge of His will for us and the power to carry that out.
12. Having had a spiritual awakening as the result of these steps, and we tried to carry this message to alcoholics and

people with eating disorders, to practice these principles in all our affairs.

Through the written exercises at the end of each chapter, you have started to piece together your big picture of yourself. We have challenged the lies of your addictions. Your work is to continue the challenge. Do be kind to and forgiving of yourself while you are in this process. If you are hateful to yourself, the addictions will come slipping through the back door to relieve the pain you are in.

We have also addressed the family. Every family situation is unique and every family's story is worth telling. We hope that you will have the blessing of being able to do family work directly. Deceased family members work can, as we mentioned, be done to an empty chair. If your family is not able or willing to do the work, the work can still be done. Be aware that if you feel sorry for yourself because your family won't participate, you re-open the door to your eating disorder and chemical abuse. Your addictions definitely will help you feel sorry for yourself and will want you to feel better by using just this once.

Your reading and writing have provided you with tools to help you recover from these devastating diseases. These tools have helped thousands of other dually-addicted women get into recovery.

We have also shared some of who we are and our struggles with eating disorders and alcohol and drug abuse. We are on this journey together and we want you to experience the daily miracles of living in recovery, to be fully engaged in the present moment, and to look forward to tomorrow with expectations that we will be blessed every day. We also know that the process of getting honest with ourselves is the hardest work any of us will ever do. We believe that you don't have to do this alone and that the women further down the road of recovery will reach back and inspire you every time you ask for their wisdom, every time you suit up and show up for a meeting, every time you say to a newcomer in a meeting, "I am glad you are here. Keep coming back."

Your own story may begin like the many patients whose voices you will hear in the next few pages. How you choose to share your story is entirely up to you, but remember: It's about giving back and knowing that your storytelling will help someone else.

IT WAS A BUSY workday in March when the phone was handed to me, "Hello, this is Sandy."

"Hello Sandy, this is Ruth, and I want to come and tell my story."

Thus began the completion of the circle of women returning to the aftercare group treatment to share their recovery stories in the aftercare group with women struggling to begin the recovery journey. Some of their stories started like this:

"My name is Mary, and I am bulimic and alcoholic. Cathy got me to go to AA, and that is where my recovery started. I didn't get my eating disorder under control until I went to OA two years later."

"My name is Carol and I am an anorexic and a meth abuser. The first person I met was Sandy. I told her that I had eaten breakfast and she didn't believe me. No, I guess she didn't believe me, given that I have an eating disorder and the way an addict lies about everything. That first meal was my losing all control of my food. And of course, I didn't have my friendly little helper. They found my stash of meth hidden in a talcum powder container."

"My name is Pearl, and I am anorexic and a laxative abuser and self- mutilator. I knew that I was going to die. I didn't want to die. I was so ready, I told myself. I also had no idea what the detox from laxatives would look like. I had so much fluid build up that I could barely walk. My bowels had no idea how to work without the massive amounts of laxatives. My life is so different now. Let me tell you how I did it."

One evening, I was thinking about our discovery of the chemical and eating disorder connection. I was recalling a recent surprise visit from a patient who had been in recovery for some time. Adrianne came up to the hospital to share her good news of recovery from cocaine. She was so proud that she had two years recovery from her addictions. At the time of her treatment, I didn't connect an eating disorder with her chemical addiction because she really minimized her thinness and chalked it up with the hazards of her profession. I wanted to give her a call to see if she would speak to my family group meeting on Thursday evening.

"Hello Adrianne, this is Cathy Napier, and I was wondering if you would speak to my family/patient group meeting in two weeks to tell your story of addiction and recovery."

"I don't know, Cathy. I haven't really told my story to anyone, but I realize that it's necessary in order to maintain recovery. I have a show in Paris next week, so when I get back I will consider coming to the group."

Adrianne called and told me she would come and tell her story if she did not have to use her real name. She wasn't ready to have the press pursue her while she was at the top of her game. I agreed that she needed to keep her anonymity.

Adrianne showed up at the group meeting, a stunning, beautiful, successful model trying to remain incognito. Her very presence took command of the room. Everyone stared as she took her seat among the crowd. When it was time to introduce her, I introduced her only as a former patient of mine, which was true. I had not seen her professionally in a few years, but she did stay in touch with me to let me know that she was working a strong program of recovery.

Adrianne took the podium to speak: "Hello, I am a cocaine addict, who used cocaine in order to maintain my weight. You see, in my profession, gaining weight means that I don't work. I'm a professional model. My story begins in childhood when I was encouraged by everyone to go into modeling because of my tall, lanky frame. Anytime I gained a few pounds, I would start to exercise or use over-the-counter diet supplements. I soon got my first big break in the modeling industry and was well on my way to becoming a 'super model,' or at least so I thought. Cocaine was rampant in the modeling and fashion industry. There was rarely a party without cocaine flowing freely.

"I remember buying the first gram on my own without having a party to attend. The cabby pulled up along the curb in a dingy part of New York, 'Please wait for me,' I said to the driver as I got out of the back seat. 'I'll only be a few minutes.' I was to meet this man that I had never seen before, but was instructed on who I should be looking for. In the distance, I could see him coming from behind two old brick buildings. I was telling myself, don't go through with this, but it seemed as if my body was not listening to the storm within my mind. I justified the use as something that would keep me within the right weight range and keep me working. The butterflies in the pit of my stomach and chest were overpowering as he approached me. He asked, 'You here to see me? Yes. Do you have the money with you?' I pulled out a wad of bills and handed it to this total stranger. This is truly insanity. He handed me a brown bag folded over several times and I put it in my purse as if I were putting in my make-up bag.

"I walked as fast as I could to the cab and told the driver to take me back to my Manhattan apartment. I nodded to the doorman and couldn't look him in the eye, thinking that he somehow knew exactly what I'd been doing. This is paranoid insanity that comes with the territory of addiction. I rushed to the elevator and could hardly get inside my apartment before I opened up the brown bag. Inside was the ingredient that would take me on a nightmare ride for the next 48 hours. I couldn't get away from my dining room table and the mirror that I used to make my line while I snorted my brains out for the next two days. I called old and new friends and tried to keep them on the phone while I was high. Food and water were something I had no interest in. The crash came only because I had no more coke left and was too exhausted to think about venturing out again. I crashed and slept for 24 straight hours. I ditched the show in Milan and, in order to forget my big mess up, I made the phone call to score again, again and again.

"I graduated to freebasing coke. I would always say, 'I will never smoke that stuff or use a needle.' Never say Never. I soon found out that freebasing makes the high, higher. I would smoke and feel like the top of my head was coming off.

"One evening, I had invited a few friends over to have a dinner party. We didn't touch the food that I had catered, but instead passed the pipe around and smoked crack all evening. When the crack was gone, we found ourselves on the floor combing through the carpet looking for more. I had long fingernails and was raking the carpet with them, hoping that we had dropped a rock. Here I was, a top model who hadn't worked in months, combing the carpet with my nails until my fingertips were raw, looking for a rock.

"Again, I crashed for days, and the depression was unbearable. I called a friend in the modeling business and told her I needed help. I knew she had been to rehab, and I needed someone to help me. I was on the road to hell with no exit sign. She gave me Cathy's phone number, and I entered treatment for my cocaine addiction and eating disorder. I had not realized that the eating disorder had triggered my cocaine addiction, so I soon ended up with two addictions to work on together.

"I stand before you today to say that I am in recovery now for three years. I eat three meals a day and a snack. I exercise with my trainer and get the proper amount of rest. I can never forget where I've been. I have to work the 12 Steps of the AA program in order to keep my recovery. I guess you could say that I now have become a storyteller."

THESE PATIENTS RETURNING TO tell their stories are the fruit of our belief in treating eating disorders and alcohol and drug abuse in a simultaneous, integrated treatment approach.

The 12th Step that we talked about comes in to play here also: "To stay sober and eating-disorder free, I have to give back." These brave women of recovery came back to share their experience, strength, and hope. The women in early recovery, or down the road in recovery, or those deciding if they want to be in recovery, relate so much to the speakers. The speakers' stories are their stories, and they have common themes, but they are also unique in that there are different roads to the same freedom that come with recovery.

# Assignment for Chapter Eight

## PSALM 139:1

My journey and my rest you scrutinize;
With all my ways you are familiar.

## *Quote*

> Everything an Indian does is in a circle, and that is because the power of the world always works in circles, and everything tries to be round.

Black Elk (1863-1950), from *Black Elk Speaks* by John G. Neihardt Meditate and reflect on the Psalm or Black Elk's quote

## Questions to Answer

1. What is the one thing you heard that spoke to your heart and made sense to you about getting into recovery?
2. What is the one thing that you wish someone would have said to you about early recover?
3. What were the most helpful tools you used? What tools do you still use?
4. Describe the benefits of recovery in your life.
5. If you had a gift to give the women who are going to read your story, what would it be?
6. What revelations have you received from writing your story?
7. How will you want to give back after you've obtained substantial recovery?

## Commentary

THIS IS OUR INVITATION to you, women of recovery: become storytellers and pass on your stories to the women who need to hear the words of your recovery. We invited you to write out the questions at the end of the chapters and to compose your unique story. We encourage you to e-mail us your stories. We will listen and we will write a second book about your stories of recovery. We have written one book about ourselves and our patients. We have described how to get into recovery and how hard the work can be to stay in recovery. Tell us how you got out of the vicious cycle of eating disorders and/or substance abuse and we will listen. There are women coming behind you who are waiting for your story. We want your story to come full circle.

GODSPEED

# Bibliography


Bartlett, John. 2002. *Bartlett's Familiar Quotations: A Collection of Passages, Phrases, and Proverbs Traced to Their Sources in Ancient and Modern Literature.* 17th ed. Edited by Justin Kaplan. Boston: Little, Brown and Company.

de Beauvoir, Simone. 2002. *The Second Sex.* Quoted in John Bartlett, *Bartlett's Familiar Quotations: A Collection of Passages, Phrases, and Proverbs Traced to Their Sources in Ancient and Modern Literature.* Boston: Little, Brown and Company.

James, Alice. 1999. *Diary entry on November 19, 1889.* Lebonon: Northeastern University Press, University Press of New England.

Jung, Carl. 1938. *Psychological Reflections: A Jung Anthology, Collected Works, Vol. 9.* Quoted in John Bartlett, *Bartlett's Familiar Quotations: A Collection of Passages, Phrases, and Proverbs Traced to Their Sources in Ancient and Modern Literature* Boston: Little, Brown and Company.

Merton, Thomas. *Thoughts in Solitude.* Rosetta Books, 2005.

Niehardt, John. Quoted in *Black Elk Speaks.* University of Nebraska Press, 1961.

Roberts, Elizabeth., and Elias, Amidon, eds. 1999. *Prayers for a Thousand Years: Blessings and Expressions of Hope for the New Millennium.* New York: HarperCollins Publishers.

Scofield, Rev. C.I. 1909. *The Holy Bible, Authorized King James Version. The Scofield Reference Bible.* New York: Oxford University Press.

Wilde, Oscar. *The Ballad of Reading Goal.* Quoted in John Bartlett, *Bartlett's Familiar Quotations: A Collection of Passages, Phrases, and Proverbs Traced to Their Sources in Ancient and Modern Literature.* Boston: Little, Brown and Company, 2002.

Wilson, Bill and Smith, Bob. The Big Book of Alcoholics Anonymous. Alcoholics Anonymous World, Inc. 2001.

# About the Authors

Sandy Mullen was a member of the Peace Corp in Iran for two years after obtaining her R.N. degree. Sandy is also a Licensed Chemical Dependency Counselor for the state of Texas. Sandy recently retired, after 11 years, from Presbyterian Hospital of Dallas where she worked as a charge nurse and program coordinator for the eating disorder unit. Prior to Sandy's work at Presbyterian Hospital, she worked as a staff nurse for nine years at Baylor Medical Center in the eating disorder program. Sandy has worked in Psychiatric nursing for a total of 32 years. Sandy currently is working at Presbyterian Hospital of Dallas as a consultant on the eating disorder unit.

Catherine (Cathy) Napier received her Bachelor's degree from Dallas Baptist University in Dallas, Texas and her Master's degree in counseling from Texas Christian University in Fort Worth, Texas. Cathy attended Rutgers University in New Brunswick, New Jersey for her post graduate studies in addiction. Cathy has worked in some of the major psychiatric hospitals in the Dallas/Fort Worth area. Cathy left Presbyterian Hospital of Dallas, where she was Director of the Chemical Dependency Program, in 2003 to work under Governor Bill Richardson's administration in Santa Fe, New Mexico. Cathy was director of the Temporary Assistance for Needy Families (TANF) substance abuse programs for the state of New Mexico for two years. Cathy is currently the founder of Operation Mother Hen and the Employee Assistance Manager for Behavioral Health Services for the Burlington Northern Santa Fe Railroad's Southwest Division.

CPSIA information can be obtained
at www.ICGtesting.com
Printed in the USA
FFOW01n1914140417
34495FF

9 781592 997978